CANDIDA-RELATED COMPLEX

CANDIDA-RELATED COMPLEX

What Your Doctor Might Be Missing

Christine Winderlin
With Keith Sehnert, M.D.

TAYLOR PUBLISHING COMPANY
Dallas, Texas

For Tristan and TJ, who taught me that even though life may end, love always endures. This book, and everything, is done in loving memory of them and the examples they provided.

Published by Taylor Publishing Company
1550 West Mockingbird Lane
Dallas, Texas 75235

Library of Congress Cataloging-in-Publication Data

Winderlin, Christine A.
Candida-related complex: what your doctor might be missing /
Christine Winderlin, with Keith W. Sehnert.
p.   cm.
Includes bibliographical references and index.
ISBN 0-87833-935-3
1. Candidiasis—Popular works.   I. Sehnert, Keith W.   II. Title.
RC123.C3W54   1996
616.9'69—dc20   96-11967
CIP

Printed in the United States of America

10   9   8   7   6   5   4   3   2   1

The treatments outlined in this book are not intended as medical advice or to replace the care of a medical professional. You should consult your doctor before undergoing any therapies, including those described in this text.

Contents

Acknowledgments

I would like to offer my heartfelt thanks to the friends and family who never stopped believing in me: Heather Burling, Tara Reeser, Katharine Winderlin, Patrick Winderlin, Susan Searles, Dawn Riordan, Ronald Pittman, and Brian Brimmer. I would also like to thank the many patients who generously gave me their time and confidence.

Introduction

When Christine Winderlin asked me to work with her on this book, to review it from a medical perspective and to add some clinical pearls I have picked up in treating nearly four thousand patients diagnosed with Candida-Related Complex (CRC), I immediately and enthusiastically agreed.

The reason for my prompt reply is captured in the last six words of the book's title, *What Your Doctor Might Be Missing*. Those few words make me sad. But even more to the point, they make me mad.

Far too many doctors are unaware of the modern epidemic of Candida infections that has spread across our country due to antibiotic overuse and abuse, ruining the health of hundreds of thousands of their patients. When you add other prescriptions, such as birth control pills, common estrogen and progesterone products used in hormone-replacement therapy, and corticosteroids and anti-inflammatory products in general, a tidal wave of doctor-caused illnesses surfaces.

What then happens—after months, years, or decades of suffering—is that these patients often undergo another type of suffering right in the doctor's office. After they go to their doctors with hope for help, their complaints are often dismissed or trivialized because their doctors are unfamiliar with CRC. Given this lack of knowledge in the medical community, it can be difficult to get the right professional help. However, with the information offered in the resource section of this book, on the Internet, from Dr. Crook's International Health Foundation, and from the Candida and Dysbiosis Foundation, helpful doctors can be identified and contacted.

Change is occurring. It may seem slow, but it is happening. As I state in my upcoming book, *The Secret Seven: Things Your Doctors Miss . . . That You Should Know,* there is a concept called a paradigm shift. A paradigm is a fixed arrangement of assumptions used to solve a condition or common problem. Sometimes when changes occur or new discoveries are made, they challenge these basic assumptions. In order for the new idea to be accepted, there must be a paradigm shift—a change in the whole way we look at things.

Historians report that paradigm shifts do not occur suddenly. It often takes twenty-five to thirty years (a generation) or more for the change to take place. One example is the case of Dr. Ignaz Semmelweiss (1818-1865), an obstetrician in Vienna, who observed that if he washed his hands and wore a clean apron over his street clothes when he delivered babies, the incidence of childbirth fever dropped dramatically to zero. (This was a major improvement, because at that time in Austria ten out of every one hundred young mothers died from these infections.)

Despite his good advice, the other doctors took no interest in adopting this simple precautionary measure. Instead, they jeered at him and said, in effect, "Our dirty hands have nothing to do with this. The reason they die is that they are evil and the Lord is taking them!"

He wrote his book, *The Etiology and Prophylaxis of Childbirth Fever,* in 1860. However, it took nearly fifty years—until World War I in 1914—before surgeons washed their hands and wore surgical gowns on a regular basis. The delay was caused not only because people had to accept the fact that childbirth fever could be caused by dirty hands, but because their whole concept of what caused disease was challenged.

With that brief step back into history we are reminded of modern times and the reluctance of today's doctors to understand CRC. When patients ask me why doctors have such difficulty accepting CRC, I give them the following explanations:

Point 1. Doctors didn't learn about CRC in medical school. And to some modern-day skeptics, if it wasn't taught ten, twenty, or thirty years ago, it doesn't exist today.

Point 2. Doctors have had little or no personal or professional exposure to the problem during their careers. In the judgment of some doctors, CRC is rare and inconsequential. As a result, many doctors have not taken the time to become informed.

Point 3. CRC symptoms are so diverse they don't fit into a simple diagnostic pattern. When you consider the wide variety of symptoms, ranging from sinus infections, gastrointestinal problems, and immune disturbances to mental complaints such as depression and "brain fog," it's not surprising that many doctors are overwhelmed at the prospect of having to make a diagnosis. They may even assume that such patients' illnesses are all in their heads.

Point 4. There is a clash of authority. Many physicians prefer a doctor-patient relationship in which they alone are the decision-makers. When aggressive patients start suggesting that they know more about their problem than their doctors (after studying about it in an article or book), some doctors may get defensive. Instead of taking the opportunity to learn from their patients, they may dismiss the whole idea or even respond with negative comments.

Despite this reluctance to change and accept new ideas, however, change will occur. This book and the knowledge about Candida that preceded it will make a difference. Patients will read it and become better informed. Their families and friends will read it and learn to support them. Parents will make better decisions for their children's health. Doctors will begin to see and understand. We will be wiser. Change will occur.

In the case of CRC, the generation (twenty-five to thirty years) of slow acceptance has passed. The Japanese researcher Dr. Iwata wrote his first article in 1970. Dr. Crook wrote his classic, *The Yeast Connection*, in 1982. Dr. Truss wrote *The Missing Diagnosis* in 1983.

It is my firm conviction that this medical paradigm is on the verge of shifting. Read this book. Help the change reach its completion. It's about time. Join us.

Keith W. Sehnert, M.D.

ALL ABOUT CANDIDA
AND CRC

—1—

What Is Going On?

Health is not valued until sickness comes along.
— Spanish proverb

The discovery of the role Candida plays in chronic illness has provided the answer to thousands of people who suffer from symptoms that range from aggravating discomforts to debilitating illnesses, and which are unexplainable in the context of traditional medical knowledge. Some have already pinpointed Candida-Related Complex (CRC) as the cause of their health troubles and have found hope and relief in the treatment of it. Reliable information on this subject, however, remains difficult to find, and many continue to suffer without the knowledge to even name their pain. Faced with mysterious symptoms and puzzled or skeptical physicians, many patients feel confusion and self-doubt. They wonder: Is this all in my head? Am I exaggerating my symptoms? If this is a real health problem, why can't I get help?

Unfortunately, CRC has not yet been recognized by a large part of the medical community because, like many other illnesses, it has yet to be fully understood. Although it is important this medical condition gain widespread recognition, it is more important that the individual patients who are suffering in silence have the information and access to treatment they need to get well and that, through public education of what causes CRC, potential cases be stopped before they even occur. Fortunately, some professionals in the medical community do treat CRC, and they have developed effective treatments

1

in recent years. No one summarizes both the controversy and the feelings of the doctors who treat CRC more passionately than Dennis Remington, M.D., and Barbara Higa, R.D., in their book *Back to Health*:

> The current concepts [about CRC] mainly arrive from attempts to explain the improvements repeatedly observed in patients who undergo therapy for suspected CC [chronic candidiasis]. Whether these attempted explanations are correct or not matters very little. They are based on currently accepted medical theories, and if some of these theories are incorrect, then the concepts will also be proven to be incorrect. The most important issue is this: thousands of doctors from around the world have treated millions of people suspected of having CC with a multi-faceted treatment program. A great number of health problems often clear up completely and dramatically.

CRC is a real illness and will no doubt eventually be fully recognized by the general medical community. Medical evidence exists even now, and more and more physicians learn about it every day, usually from patients in their care. As more documentation and other evidence point to Candida as the cause of a diverse list of symptoms, and as more patients respond positively to treatments, the interest in research in this area will grow, and those who suffer from CRC will receive the support and affirmation they deserve. But more importantly, they will get relief from symptoms and return to health at last.

Making Sense of CRC

CRC is a medical condition that occurs when an organism commonly found in all of our bodies multiplies out of control. The organism is called *Candida albicans* (pronounced kan´did-a al´bi-kans), though it is often referred to simply as Candida.

Many questions and much confusion surround CRC, and several names have been used to describe Candida infection over the years. The chronic illness discussed in this book, however, will be called Candida-Related Complex, or CRC, because other related health problems such as allergies, food sensitivities, hormone dysfunction, environmental sensitivities, hypoglycemia, and stress-related disorders are often present.

CRC describes an illness that can have any one of hundreds of possible symptoms. It is not fatal and can be brought under control with the help of a special diet and medication.

In an effort to be as accurate as possible, sometimes the phrase "Candida-related illness" or "Candida-related problems" will be used. These phrases describe a situation in which Candida is negatively affecting an individual's health, but the individual doesn't necessarily have full-blown CRC. An example might be a child who suffers from hyperactivity, learning disabilities, or autism induced by Candida, but who exhibits no other symptoms associated with CRC.

Making sense of Candida-related problems is like putting together a jigsaw puzzle. You can solve the problem only bit by bit, connecting one piece at a time. Gradually, the picture becomes clearer and clearer. Eventually you will see the whole image, but the process can be difficult, time-consuming, and frustrating.

Managing Candida is probably unlike anything you've ever done before. It requires a new way of thinking. We are accustomed to medical problems such as diseases that *invade* our bodies, but Candida *already exists* inside each one of us. When we are healthy, our immune systems regulate its growth, and it is harmless. If it is allowed to multiply unchecked in our bodies, however, it can cause serious problems.

Although CRC has not yet been universally accepted, Candida has long been known by physicians and scientists to cause other diseases. Any infection by Candida is called candidiasis. Two types of candidiasis have been established and widely addressed in medical journals: superficial candidiasis and systemic candidiasis. In fact, thousands of medical journal articles have been written about Candida's unique effect on the body. All types of Candida infections occur when the patient's immune defenses have been damaged by factors such as heavy use of antibiotics, environmental chemical overload, or a serious illness. One important point to keep in mind is that the Candida organism can take advantage of only a body that has weakened immune defenses.

Superficial candidiasis describes localized yeast infection of the skin and mucous membranes. Two examples are vaginitis and oral thrush. Although much is known about this superficial candidiasis, it is frequently considered a nuisance rather than a serious or debilitating disease. However, superficial Candida infections that are recurring and difficult to treat are often symptoms of more serious Candida-related problems.

Systemic candidiasis, also known as "deep candidiasis," is serious and life threatening. Unlike superficial candidiasis, it is almost never related to CRC. Systemic candidiasis describes a Candida infection of one or more surfaces or internal organs and affects patients who have been immunocompromised. Although the term *immunocompromised* has a wide range of use and can apply to anyone with a deficient immune system, in this case it refers only to those individuals whose immune systems have been fully compromised by a debilitating condition such as cancer or AIDS. Systemic candidiasis occurs when Candida disseminates throughout the body. This siege of the body by Candida differs from the dissemination of Candida by-products throughout the bloodstream, which is typical of CRC.

Both superficial and systemic candidiasis are recognized by the medical community, so at least some of the dangers the Candida organism poses have already been acknowledged. And, considering the vast number of people who exhibit signs of CRC, it can be only a matter of time before it, too, is widely accepted as a legitimate disorder to be treated regularly by general practitioners.

Sarah's Story

I first heard about CRC through a woman whose eighteen-year-old daughter, Sarah, was having bizarre and seemingly unexplainable medical problems that started after she began taking birth control pills. Neither mother nor daughter knew what was causing Sarah's problems or what to do about them.

The most frightening and potentially dangerous of Sarah's symptoms were the ovarian cysts she developed every month. One week after she discontinued birth control pills, a cyst in one of her ovaries ruptured. Since then Sarah has had a total of seven cysts rupture. "At the time, I had abdominal pain that my doctor said was probably nothing," she said. Sarah developed a cyst the second half of her menstrual cycle every month that would either rupture or be absorbed back into her body.

The cysts were not only extremely painful, but also life threatening. If they ruptured, they could cut off the blood supply to Sarah's ovaries. The result would be hemorrhaging, which is the loss of a large amount of blood during a short period of time, and Sarah could need emergency surgery. Besides ovarian cysts, her other symptoms were depression, fatigue, irritability, migraine headaches, blurred vision, and severe leg and chest pains. Sarah also had recurring vaginal and urinary tract infections.

Sarah and her mother were at a loss for what to do. The doctors they consulted dismissed Sarah's problems as stress-related, irrelevant, or psychosomatic. "The doctors connected my problems with the pill to stress. If the doctors didn't know what my problem was they dismissed it as untreatable. After I went back, still sick, my doctors were intimidated," Sarah said.

Although Sarah's symptoms, particularly the ovarian cysts, were more dramatic than most CRC patients, Sarah's medical history is a textbook example of CRC. Not only had Sarah been prescribed antibiotics for colds and flus, but she also took birth control pills and consumed a high-sugar diet. As a freshman in college, Sarah started taking birth control pills to reduce her painful menstrual cramps. During high school her physician frequently prescribed antibiotics for upper respiratory infections. "My doctor handed them [antibiotics] to me like candy," she said. Despite her mother's urgings to eat nutritious food, Sarah didn't listen and lived from one sugar high to the next. "My motto always was: Why have a salad when I could eat dessert?" she joked.

After Sarah suffered one year of pain and uncertainty, a relative suggested she pick up a book on *Candida albicans*. "I was elated when we found out it was Candida. I didn't care what the treatment would be, I was just thrilled to put a name to my problem and to find out that there could be a possible cure," Sarah said.

Since then Sarah has begun the slow recovery process. Through a list found in the back of the book on Candida, she found a doctor in her area and immediately began taking medications and went on a special diet designed to check Candida growth: "If I eat sugar now, I'm in pain. My body just can't handle it," Sarah explained.

Two years later she is much better, but still battling several medical problems including endometriosis, which is another commonly reported problem related to CRC. Looking back on her experiences, she is relieved that she was able to find out what was wrong. "What means the most to me now is that I no longer have emotional problems and mood swings," she said.

What Sarah went through was terrifying, not just for her, but for her entire family. I know because Sarah is my sister, and I shared my mother's grief, confusion, and frustration as Sarah's repeated attempts to escape her pain failed again and again.

Sarah, like many others with CRC, suffered needlessly before receiving treatment simply because no one bothered to help her. None of her doctors had heard of CRC. When they couldn't fit her symptoms into easily defined categories, her doctors dismissed them. Since the solution wasn't a simple prescription, they didn't want to be bothered with her.

And even now her choice of doctors is limited because many doctors remain uneducated about this medical problem. The majority of physicians are either unfamiliar with CRC or, because the myriad and complex symptoms make it difficult to fit into a traditional disease pattern, they are unwilling to consider the possibility that it exists. This makes treatment costly because medical insurance frequently doesn't cover treatments. And when Sarah was able to put a name to her strange medical problem, doctors were reluctant to help her because she diagnosed the problem from a book she bought in a bookstore.

Although Sarah's health is much improved, many other patients are experiencing symptoms and are not being helped by the medical community. One reason is because the medications that contribute to CRC have been mainstays in health-care treatment for decades. The primary contributors to CRC are birth control pills, antibiotics, and prednisone and other anti-inflammatory medications. Accepting these medications as contributors to a harmful health condition would require radical rethinking on the part of the medical community. Even though information about CRC and supporting medical evidence have been available for twenty years, the controversy remains. But as more and more people experience symptoms and demand help from mainstream medical professionals, current thinking will continue to be challenged until CRC is accepted in the medical community.

—2—

What Is Candida-Related Complex?

Knowledge is a process of piling up facts;
wisdom lies in their simplification.
—Martin H. Fischer in *Fischerisms*,
by Howard Fabing and Ray Marr

Although an estimated 80 to 90 percent of CRC sufferers are women of childbearing age, the illness also affects men and children. The most common symptoms that appear in women, however, differ from those seen most often in men, and those occurring frequently in children are different from both of these. In addition, CRC's diverse symptoms may vary from person to person. For example, one woman might suffer leg pains, depression, and severe migraine headaches while another has abdominal pain, food allergies, and memory loss. The fact that Candida causes different reactions in the people it affects and can be related to other conditions, such as allergies, depression, and chemical sensitivities, is a major reason CRC hasn't been accepted by much of the medical community.

Often a disease or illness has easily recognizable signs or symptoms. One example of a disease that fits into a neat diagnostic package is chicken pox. Physicians are familiar with chicken pox and have been treating it for centuries. They know chicken pox begins with a slight fever and that itchy poxes generally develop first on the back and chest. Physicians learned about chicken pox in medical school and know what causes it, whom it primarily affects, and how to treat it. When confronted with an illness that isn't as easily definable, doctors have a more difficult time naming the cause. And if a patient exhibits very complex and seemingly unrelated symptoms, physicians may even decline to make a diagnosis or assume the problems are caused by unresolved mental problems.

CRC isn't easy to pigeonhole or classify, and conventional medicine has been reluctant to recognize it. Understandably, physicians find it hard to believe that anything can affect every system of the body. Yet Candida does. William G. Crook, M.D., the most widely published author on Candida and yeast-related health problems, says, "There is a general saying: If a physician is not up on something, he's down on it. Physicians will initially reject something because they don't know anything about it." Dr. Crook is author of the best-selling *The Yeast Connection* and *The Yeast Connection and the Woman*.

CRC is different from other medical conditions in that its symptoms vary from person to person. Because it is a very individual condition with seemingly unconnected symptoms, patients often become puzzled and alarmed. Like physicians, they are accustomed to fitting symptoms together to form a neat and logical picture. Treating Candida-related problems successfully requires a new way of thinking by both patients and physicians.

Although CRC is caused by *Candida albicans,* which is a usually harmless yeast organism, the real problem is what allows the microorganism to grow out of control. One of the main contributors is a weak immune system. Some things that can weaken the immune system are nutritional deficiencies, infection, emotional stress, environmental chemicals and pollutants, and environmental molds. Cornell University Medical College Associate Research Professor Steven Witkin, Ph.D., notes that whether the body clears itself of Candida depends on the cellular immune system. A weak immune system will succumb to Candida and a strong one will not: "Since an intact cellular immune system is essential for defending against fungal infections, it is not surprising that factors leading to alterations in components of this system also predispose one to *Candida* infections."

Other important contributors to Candida growth are broad-spectrum antibiotics, birth control pills, a diet high in sugar and junk food, steroids, and cortisone and other drugs. In different ways, all of these factors increase the production of Candida, which then gives off toxins and causes a wide variety of health problems.

Sometimes CRC appears immediately after the use of antibiotics or any of the above mentioned factors that can spur Candida-related problems. According to Dr. Dennis Remington, coauthor of *Back to Health,* however, it is more likely that CRC will develop gradually, "with symptoms increasing in number and severity over a period of time."

Candida is a yeast organism, and yeasts are a subgroup of a family of fungi. Fungi, including yeasts, are thought to cause disease mainly in plants, while bacteria are thought to cause disease in animals, including humans. Given this, it is easy to understand why so much of medicine is devoted to fighting bacteria and *not* fungi. To most health professionals, bacteria pose a greater threat to human health than fungi, or yeasts. While the medical focus on bacteria is necessary, it takes attention away from the equally serious health threat of fungal infections. And treating medical conditions caused by complex organisms like yeasts and other fungi in the same way bacterial infections are treated isn't effective at all. A better understanding of fungal infections and their increasing effect on human health would improve health and lessen the mystery and prevalence of some chronic illnesses.

Because Candida has long been considered harmless, it is hard for many physicians to now believe it can cause serious problems. For them, Candida's role in human health is limited to the two obvious Candida infections mentioned previously. C. Orian Truss, M.D., a Birmingham internist and allergist, was the first to establish a link between Candida and more general human illnesses. He emphasizes that because Candida's role in human health has long been seen as firmly established, it is hard for doctors to now think of it as causing chronic symptoms. He writes:

> The very fact of its universal presence [in most humans] probably accounts in large part for the neglect in attempting to relate this yeast to serious disease. Instead, it is today relegated to the role of an aggravating nuisance when it infects mucous membranes, skin, and nails; the one exception is the rare septicemic dissemination in the chronically ill, often immunocompromised host.

As Dr. Truss mentions, Candida's presence is easily detectable in superficial infections like diaper rash or thrush, or as a complication in serious illnesses like cancer and AIDS. It is far harder to pin down Candida as a cause of chronic illness. As Dr. Truss notes, "Less well recognized has been the great harm that may be done by products released chronically into the bloodstream when this yeast succeeds in establishing itself in the tissues."

It is also because Candida has always been seen as unimportant that the crucial issue of how antibiotics influence Candida was (and still is) largely ignored by practicing physicians. Since antibiotics are generally accepted as one of the leading contributors to Candida growth and the development of CRC, to miss the connection between Candida and chronic illness is two times a tragedy. According to Mildred Seelig, M.D., author of a definitive medical journal article on antibiotics and Candida, "Because of the widespread assumption that only rarely is *C. albicans* the cause of disease, and then only in debilitated patients, its outgrowth on the administration of antibiotics has often been deemed of little importance." In her article, Dr. Seelig presents proof that the pathogenicity of Candida is "markedly increased in the presence of factors that impair host resistance." The goal of the physicians who treat this complex illness is to have CRC accepted as a valid illness and also to establish the role that the Candida organism plays in chronic illness so that people who are suffering from it can be properly treated.

Do You Have CRC?

This questionnaire is provided as a guide for you and your physician. It is designed for adults, not children.

Have you ever taken broad-spectrum antibiotics for prolonged periods of time? (one course for about two months or longer, or several short courses of antibiotics during a short time period)   yes ☐   no ☐

Have you ever taken cortisone medications for long periods of time?   yes ☐   no ☐

Have you ever taken birth control pills?   yes ☐   no ☐

Do you frequently eat foods that contain large amounts of sugar?   yes ☐   no ☐

Do you crave foods that contain sugar, yeast, or alcohol?   yes ☐   no ☐

Do certain foods or chemicals provoke allergic reactions?   yes ☐   no ☐

Do you feel terrible all over and no treatments have helped you?   yes ☐   no ☐

Do your symptoms worsen in moldy places?   yes ☐   no ☐

Do your symptoms worsen on damp, muggy days?   yes ☐   no ☐

Do your symptoms worsen around tobacco smoke, perfume, gasoline, or other chemical smells?   yes ☐   no ☐

Do you have frequent infections or skin problems?   yes ☐   no ☐

Do you frequently have vaginal infections or other problems such as vaginal burning, itching, or discharge? Have you ever had trouble becoming pregnant?   yes ☐   no ☐

Do you have PMS or other menstrual problems?   yes ☐   no ☐

Have you lost interest in sex or become impotent?   yes ☐   no ☐

Do you have frequent gastrointestinal disturbances such as bloating, constipation, heartburn, indigestion, or gas?   yes ☐   no ☐

Do you frequently have emotional and mental symptoms such as irritability, depression, mood swings, anxiety, agitation, or nervousness?   yes ☐   no ☐

Do you ever have trouble concentrating or feel disoriented or spacy?   yes ☐   no ☐

Do you commonly have symptoms such as severe leg pains, frequent headaches, muscle aches, chest pains, dizziness, or recurring kidney or bladder infections?   yes ☐   no ☐

If you answered "yes" to four or five questions, you may have CRC. Six or seven "yes" answers means you probably have CRC. Eight or nine "yes" answers indicates you most likely have CRC.

Symptoms Associated with Candida

The Candida organism can affect all nine systems of the body: digestive, nervous, cardiovascular, lymphatic, respiratory, reproductive, urinary, endocrine, and musculoskeletal. The toxins secreted by Candida affect each system and each system affects the others. While it may seem odd to say all of the systems of the body can be affected by one organism, it makes more sense when you remember every part of your body is connected to every other part.

A full listing of the symptoms of CRC is extremely important for two reasons. The symptoms not only characterize the illness, but are also a part of the patient's medical history that doctors use as a basis for their diagnosis. Although the symptoms vary from person to person, several symptoms are much more commonly reported than others. Female patients diagnosed with CRC report they have feelings of unrealness fatigue, and severe depression. One problem commonly reported by women is break-through bleeding or spotting, which is an irregular blood flow that happens despite use of birth control pills. Another is sensitivity to strong smells such as chemical odors, tobacco smoke, automobile exhaust, and perfumes.

The common signals and symptoms of Candida overgrowth include, but are not limited to, the following list of ailments:

General Symptoms
fatigue
weight gain
weight loss
loss of balance
dizziness
poor coordination
insomnia
recurring ear infections
loss of appetite
overeating
pelvic pain
psoriasis
acne

Gastrointestinal System
chronic heartburn
gastritis
colitis
distention
bloating
gas
indigestion
diarrhea
rectal itching
hemorrhoids
abdominal pain
constipation

Emotional/Mental
irritability
depression
agitation
short attention span
crying spells
anxiety
nervousness
jittery behavior
lethargy
inability to concentrate
poor memory
memory loss
headaches
migraine headaches
brain fog

Women
vaginitis or vaginal discharge
endometriosis
menstrual cramping
failure to menstruate
too frequent periods
premenstrual syndrome (PMS)
problems getting pregnant
frequent miscarriages
loss of interest in sex

Men
impotence
prostatitis
jock itch
athlete's foot

Overall Body

severe leg pains
chest pains
wheezing or shortness of breath
muscle aches and pains
muscle weakness or paralysis
joint pains or stiffness
joint swelling or arthritis
poor circulation (cold hands
  and feet)

Allergic Symptoms

hay fever
chronic sinusitis
hives
asthma
allergies or sensitivities to
  chemicals and foods

Diseases or Problems Thought to Be Related to or Affected by Candida

arthritis
fungal infections such as
  athlete's foot, ringworm,
  jock itch
mitral valve prolapse
Crohn's disease
Hodgkin's disease
hypoglycemia
lupus erythematosus
scleroderma
autism
chronic respiratory disease

myasthenia gravis
alcoholism
anorexia nervosa
bulimia
multiple sclerosis
inflammatory bowel disease

Common Candida-Related Problems of Children

thrush
diaper rash
mood swings
colic
irritability
recurring ear infections
hyperactivity
learning difficulties
short attention span
nasal congestion
chronic cough/wheezing
headaches
digestive problems
constipation
diarrhea
gas and bloating
sweet cravings

Urinary System

recurring kidney and bladder
  infections
urethritis
cystitis
burning upon urination
frequent urination

Food cravings usually accompany Candida overgrowth. These include any and all forms of sugar, including white sugar, brown sugar, honey, molasses, maple syrup, and other syrups. Many people report needing or longing for foods that contain large amounts of sugar like ice cream, chocolate, desserts, soft drinks, fruit juice, fresh fruit, and dried fruit. Other frequently craved foods are yeast breads, cereal grains (oatmeal, wheat, barley, rye, millet, rice, and buckwheat) and high carbohydrate foods such as potatoes and pasta.

While the full range of symptoms varies from person to person, some symptoms are much more common than others. Leo Galland, M.D., who has treated and studied hundreds of patients with Candida-related health problems, presented summarized data on the common symptoms of ninety-one CRC patients at a recent Candida Update Conference. Dr. Galland discovered twelve common symptoms among the ninety-one patients he studied and reported the following:

- 89 percent experienced fatigue
- 86 percent experienced food intolerances
- 81 percent experienced gastrointestinal disturbances
- 71 percent experienced alcohol intolerances
- 61 percent experienced chronic vaginitis
- 55 percent experienced memory impairment
- 54 percent experienced depression
- 46 percent experienced chemical hypersensitivity
- 44 percent experienced premenstrual syndrome
- 39 percent experienced anxiety
- 29 percent experienced headaches
- 19 percent experienced carbohydrate cravings

One of the frequent criticisms of CRC concerns the symptoms, which critics say are too vague and can apply to anyone at anytime. In their book *The Yeast Syndrome*, John Parks Trowbridge, M.D., and Morton Walker, D.P.M., respond to this statement by saying, "That the disease symptoms may apply to almost all sick patients at some time is exactly the point made by those informed pioneers—the medical mavericks—who have educated themselves about the condition and regularly treat the Candida syndrome. Indications of ill health from this yeast syndrome are wide ranging."

Even though CRC isn't an easy medical condition to understand or live with, keep in mind that not only are the necessary treatments very successful in helping CRC patients, but also that most patients do regain their health.

—3—

The Candida Organism and How It Affects the Body

There is more wisdom in your body than in your deepest philosophy.
— Friedrich Nietzsche in *Human, All Too Human*, Pt. II

What is this organism that causes so many problems and how does it grow out of control? An overview of the Candida organism and the role it plays in human health will provide insight into this complex illness and help explain the necessary steps toward regaining health.

Most people think the closest they come to yeasts every day is when they consume foods like bread and beverages like beer and wine, which have been produced with the help of yeasts. Many are unaware of the role yeasts play in their everyday health. Even though they are generally undetectable to the human eye, more than three hundred types of yeast are part of the normal surface of the human skin.

And inside our bodies up to five hundred varieties of viral, bacterial, and fungal microorganisms, including Candida, exist. An estimated one hundred trillion organisms, or about one to two solid pounds, live their entire lives inside individual human bodies. Ideally they live in relative harmony and balance. Beneficial bacteria inside us, along with our immune systems, help keep Candida and other potentially harmful organisms under control. That's why antibiotics, which are designed to kill harmful bacteria but which also kill helpful bacteria, contribute to Candida infection. With the bacteria gone, our immune systems have a tougher job of battling

Candida. And if they are too weak to meet the challenge, Candida will flourish. The finely tuned harmony of our internal flora becomes unbalanced, and sickness results.

Sidney M. Baker, M.D., former director of the Gesell Institute of Human Development in New Haven, Connecticut, and former professor at the Yale School of Medicine, discusses the role of yeasts in our bodies in his pamphlet *Notes on the Yeast Problem: Essays and a Yeast Free Diet*:

> I know yeasts as seen through the microscope. They look as docile and simple as vegetables. The more I get to know the aggressive side of their chemistry, the more I think of them as animals. The more I get to know the complex way they interact with our bodies, the less I think of them as strangers, and the more I think of them as a part of us. It is especially important, in that sense, to view the yeast problem as a state of inner imbalance rather than an attack from the outside from a microbe or a disease.

Candida and the Human Body

Candida albicans lives in the mucous membranes of the mouth, intestinal tract, digestive tract, vagina, and other areas of both sick and healthy people's bodies. Because Candida is normally in our bodies, its presence doesn't necessarily indicate unwellness—that's one reason confirming CRC can be tricky. A test that comes back negative for the presence of Candida could actually indicate a problem, since the presence of some Candida is consistent with normal immune system function. C. Orian Truss, M.D., the first to discover the role yeasts play in human health, writes: "Since *Candida albicans* is in everyone, it is readily apparent that its presence is entirely compatible with a lifetime of excellent health."

Candida is the most prolific yeast organism in the human body and prefers to live in the gastrointestinal (GI) tract, which runs from mouth to rectum. Two other common residences of Candida are the genitourinary tract (where the organs responsible for reproduction and urination are located) and the female genitalia, usually the vagina. However, Candida has been known to infect every tissue in the body except hair.

As stated previously, Candida is incapable of causing harm in a healthy person and may actually perform a positive role in human health.

Dr. Shirley S. Lorenzani, author of *Candida: A Twentieth Century Disease*, describes Candida as a friend and not an enemy. She writes that Candida "signals us when drugs, foods, and other forms of distress have weakened our defenses. It is our smoke detector, our burglar alarm, our seat-belt buzzer. The signals may be annoying, but the early warning, if heeded, enables us to avoid disaster." According to Dr. Lorenzani, by acting as a barometer, Candida signals the need for a reexamination of lifestyle choices—choices that include an improper diet, little or no exercise, and the use of oral contraceptives and antibiotics that can damage the body.

Although Dr. Lorenzani makes an excellent point about Candida being an important warning signal, labeling Candida a "friend" may be putting too positive a spin on the problem. Generally speaking, though those adversely affected by Candida are no doubt grateful to have (in the long run) improved their health, the path to good health was most likely unpleasant and perhaps even extremely costly.

Candida Toxins: Poisons to Our System

Candida albicans is a very complex organism. It can injure our bodies and cause infections by penetrating the tissues of our bodies. In addition, it releases at least seventy-nine toxic chemical substances, called antigens, into our bodies. These toxins, or poisons, are responsible for many of the symptoms described previously as being characteristic of CRC. Our immune systems create antibodies to fight each toxin. Healthy immune systems can effectively battle the Candida, counteract the toxins, and maintain a balance in our bodies. When our defenses are weakened, however, the Candida and its toxins travel throughout our bodies, wreaking havoc with our health. They even attack our already impaired immune systems, weakening them further.

Two of the most detrimental Candida toxins are acetaldehyde and ethanol, both of which are poisonous to the tissues of our bodies. Other notable Candida toxins include canditoxin, mannan, proteinase, tyramine, and polysaccharide protein complexes.

Most of us are aware that when mixed together, sugar and yeast produce ethanol, a type of alcohol. The same process happens inside our bodies: the sugars we eat react with yeast, and ethanol is a byproduct. Acetaldehyde, which is used commercially to make acetic acid, drugs, and perfumes and is six times more toxic to brain tissue than ethanol, is then produced as the ethanol breaks down. Not only are ethanol and acetaldehyde generally toxic to our system, they also cause the following problems in our bodies: cell membrane defects and destruction of enzymes (which are important to digestion, respiration, and other bodily functions).

The cells primarily affected by toxins are red and white blood cells. Chemicals released by Candida make the cell membranes more rigid and less flexible, which keeps the cells from successfully carrying out their necessary functions. One of the functions of red blood cells is to carry oxygen throughout the body. To do this they have to be elastic enough to squeeze down to about one-seventh of their normal size to be able to get into the body's tiniest blood vessels, the capillaries. By making the red blood cell walls rigid, the Candida chemicals impede the flow of blood, and therefore oxygen, to all of the organs and tissues of the body. White blood cells make up part of the immune system. When their cell walls become rigid, their ability to fight off infection is decreased, leaving our bodies more susceptible to illnesses. Rigid cell walls of other cells in your body decrease their ability to absorb needed nutrients and vitamins.

Damaged cell walls also keep hormones from penetrating cells. Hormones travel throughout the body via the bloodstream, regulating body functions. One example of the effect this has on your body involves the function of the thyroid hormones, which regulate metabolism. When thyroid hormones can't enter cells, the normal metabolism of the body is slowed, causing decreased body temperature, intolerance to cold, and most importantly, fatigue. One reason this source of fatigue can't be diagnosed through laboratory tests is that blood tests measure only the amount of thyroid hormones in the blood, not their ability to perform. This is a complex topic about which entire books have been written. For more information see *Solved: The Riddle of Illness* by Stephen E. Langer, M.D.

Enzyme destruction is another problem caused by chemicals released by Candida. Enzymes are proteins produced by the cells that act as "chemical helpers" and break molecules down into usable bits and pieces. The chemicals and toxins produced by Candida can destroy enzymes, and when this happens all of the functions of the body slow down.

A 1984 article by Dr. Truss called "Metabolic Abnormalities in Patients with Chronic Candidiasis: The Acetaldehyde Hypothesis," published in the *Journal of Orthomolecular Psychiatry*, links the production of acetaldehyde in the body to some of the symptoms that characterize CRC. In the article, Dr. Truss says that the result of having this "very toxic substance" in the body is a disruption of normal cell processes and the normal intestinal absorptive processes. The toxicity of acetaldehyde has been well-established, and "The known toxic effects of acetaldehyde are more than adequate to account for all the metabolic disturbances found in the [twenty-four] patients who were subjects of this study."

What makes Dr. Truss's acetaldehyde theory so significant is that if it is correct, it would explain two of the most often cited questions about the validity of CRC. His theory would explain some of the odd symptoms of CRC and would provide a chemical mechanism that explains how Candida can simultaneously interfere with various systems and organs throughout the body. We will know more when further studies have been performed and additional evidence surfaces.

Candida and Digestion: The "Leaky Gut" Problem

Candida overgrowth in the gut, or intestine, is responsible for digestive problems and food allergies, two commonly reported symptoms of CRC. Common digestive symptoms include bloating, constipation, and gas.

In a recent issue of *Mastering Food Allergies*, Gruia Ionescu, M.D., the scientific research director of a clinic in Bavaria that specializes in allergic and degenerative diseases, discusses the importance of a healthy digestive tract and explains how Candida overgrowth contributes to allergic sensitivities. He reports that approximately half of his patients who are treated for allergies have a problem with Candida overgrowth in their intestines.

When the digestive process functions abnormally, there are both short-term and long-term effects. The short-term effects are the daily digestive problems and food allergies. The long-term effects are a bit more complex. The poor digestion and malabsorption of nutrients, in time, contribute to a dysfunctional immune system.

During digestion there is a chemical breakdown of organic molecules (by enzymes) into substances that can be used by the body. These substances then enter the bloodstream through the process of absorption that begins in the stomach. Only nutrients, which are very small molecules, are supposed to pass into circulation. When large molecules are allowed to pass into the circulating blood, digestive problems occur. The intestinal mucosa, which is the lining of the stomach and intestines, plays a very important role in either allowing or stopping molecules from passing through.

Candida weakens the intestinal mucosa and makes it more permeable, allowing the wrong molecules to pass through it. In other words the gut leaks, and large protein molecules, toxins, and food allergens are absorbed into the bloodstream. An allergen is anything that can cause an allergic reaction. Food allergens can also cause systemic and nervous system symptoms.

"When the gut contains an overgrowth of Candida, the lining becomes very inflamed—and less efficient at handling food," reported Dr. Ionescu. When a leaky gut allows undigested particles to pass into the bloodstream the immune system identifies these foreign substances as "invaders" and attacks them. When nontoxic substances are attacked in this manner the results are often allergic reactions.

The solution to the leaky gut problem and the resulting symptoms is to reduce Candida overgrowth in the body. Once the overgrowth is controlled through medications and a strict diet, the leaky gut problem will decrease and food allergies will subside. In the meantime, if you suffer from problems associated with a leaky gut, you may want to avoid other factors that exacerbate the problem. Antibiotics can interfere with the absorption of nutrients and the normal repair of the mucosa. Antacids and anti-inflammatory drugs, which include aspirin and ibuprofen, also weaken the mucosa.

Understanding that the Candida organism can affect our bodies in many ways is crucial to learning how to recover from CRC.

—4—

Who Is Affected and Why?

First the patient, second the patient, third the patient, fourth the patient, fifth the patient, and then maybe comes science. We first do everything for the patient; science can wait, research can wait.
— Béla Schick, quoted by I.J. Wolf in
Aphorisms and Facetiae of Béla Schick

Men, women, and children can all be negatively affected by Candida, but the reasons they are affected and the symptoms they experience vary greatly. And although anyone can be affected by Candida, women are more likely to develop Candida-related problems for a variety of reasons, which can be divided into two categories: factors biologically inherent to women and behaviors common to women.

Women

The typical young woman with Candida-related problems has most likely consulted many types of physicians including gynecologists, internists, urologists, otolaryngologists, and neurologists. "And because their complaints continue and no apparent explanation is found, they may be told, 'You'll just have to learn to live with these symptoms.' If they continue to complain, their families, friends, and physicians will usually label them as 'hypochondriacs,'" writes Dr. Crook.

There are several facets of a typical woman's life that happen to affect Candida growth. They include hormonal changes, birth control pills, antibiotics, the female anatomy, and pregnancy. Certain hormones cause Candida to grow and multiply and are common

21

during adolescence, normal menstrual cycles, and pregnancy. Birth control pills, which provide doses of synthetic hormones, are another common aspect of women's lives that causes hormonal levels to change and encourages yeast colonization. Not only do birth control pills disrupt the hormonal balance, they also contain progesterone, which has been found to especially stimulate the growth of Candida. As Dr. Truss notes, except prior to puberty and after menopause, a woman is repeatedly exposed to progesterone, a potent stimulus to yeast growth.

The female anatomy also works against women. Because of the structure of the female bladder system, especially the urethra, women are especially prone to cystitis and other urinary tract problems and are often given broad-spectrum antibiotics to treat these problems. In addition, the vagina's warm, moist environment provides an ideal place for Candida growth.

Furthermore, teenage women who are concerned with acne often take antibiotics like tetracycline. And since women visit doctors more often than men in general, they are more likely to receive medications that encourage yeast growth.

PMS and Candida

Premenstrual syndrome (PMS) and Candida appear to be related. Many women who suffer from PMS find that their symptoms improve dramatically when they follow a Candida control diet and medications that discourage yeast growth.

PMS has been acknowledged as a health problem only in the last decade even though an estimated twenty-five million women in the United States suffer from mood, appetite, and weight fluctuations every month. PMS is defined as physical and psychological symptoms that occur or increase during the week or so preceding menstruation. These symptoms may subside when the period starts. They frequently include painful or swollen breasts, bloating, abdominal pain, headache, and backache. Also critical are the mental and nervous system symptoms, especially depression, anxiety, irritability, and behavioral changes. Symptoms vary from woman to woman and can range from mild cramping to almost disabling pain.

There are several connections between PMS and Candida infection, which can be broken into two basic categories. The first is similar symptoms and circumstances and the second is that both PMS and CRC symptoms improve after the same therapy. Given the following evidence, it is easy to understand the possibility of a link between the two medical conditions.

Not only do CRC and PMS have similar symptoms, but during the premenstrual phase of the menstrual cycle the symptoms of CRC intensify. Both are influenced by multiple pregnancies and nutritional deficiencies, and both conditions share high frequencies of allergies. Dr. Remington notes, "Both conditions are associated with carbohydrate metabolism problems. Both are frequently associated with alcohol intolerance, sugar and sweet cravings, and low-blood-sugar symptoms, such as dizziness, weakness, and other symptoms relieved by eating."

The same therapy, a combination of diet and nutritional supplements, cures or eases both illnesses. A diet that excludes sugar has been found to be especially helpful in treating both PMS and Candida. Women who follow the diet recommended for their CRC also report that, to their surprise, their PMS symptoms have either diminished or disappeared. "Some women have reported that their menstrual period caught them unprepared—there were none of the usual unpleasant warning symptoms," writes Dr. Remington.

A 1987 article by Jay S. Schinfeld, M.D., in *The Female Patient* discusses a study that explores a possible link between PMS and Candida infection. Dr. Schinfeld conducted a controlled study with prospective subjects from the Premenstrual Syndrome Unit at the University of Tennessee College of Medicine in Memphis. All of the women selected had failed to respond to routine treatment for their severe PMS, and many also had vaginal or oral candidiasis that was either resistant to medication or resumed after medication was stopped.

Dr. Schinfeld found that a combination of yeast-free diet and medication produced relief in ten of the fifteen women. None of the women who received the yeast-free diet and medication reported worsening of her symptoms, compared to those who didn't receive medication or a specific diet. Dr. Schinfeld also said that after long-term follow-up, the symptoms most often reported by the women who didn't improve were depression, anger, and anxiety. "However, few patients receiving a yeast-elimination diet with oral or vaginal medication continued to have symptoms," added Dr. Schinfeld.

One of Dr. Schinfeld's statements neatly sums up the problems the medical community has, not just with the CRC diagnosis, but also with the treatment: "Treated patients showed significant physical and psychological improvements over untreated controls, but the mechanism for this improvement and the role of yeast in this disorder remain controversial."

Although Dr. Schinfeld's study contained a small number of subjects, his findings point toward a possible connection between Candida and PMS. In his summary, Dr. Schinfeld cautions that this therapy remains unproven until it can be tested on a larger scale. He also asserts that vulvovaginitis, pain and itching after intercourse, and in some cases mood alteration in PMS patients are responsive to the standard anti-Candida treatment of diet and medication.

Many gynecologists report using anti-Candida therapy to help patients who have PMS. Although Candida isn't the cause of PMS, Dr. Crook said "that in the patient with the characteristic history suggesting yeast-connected illness, a trial of anti-Candida therapy is warranted." He has found that a special diet, nystatin, and nutritional supplements are helpful in treating PMS.

There are several possible reasons that explain how PMS and Candida may be related. The reasons include the influence of hormones such as estrogen and progesterone and the toxins produced by the Candida organism.

Although no one knows for sure what exactly causes PMS, there are several theories. Some scientists believe PMS may be linked to too much estrogen and not enough progesterone in the body. Progesterone is a hormone that is naturally present in higher levels during the menstrual cycle. Hormonal fluctuations, which include the addition of progesterone to the body, are known to influence Candida growth and CRC. When progesterone levels are high, such as during pregnancy, during the menstrual cycle, and when synthetic hormones like birth control pills are being taken, women are more likely to develop vaginitis, which is basically a localized Candida infection.

The toxins produced by Candida may also play a part in causing or influencing PMS. Dr. Remington theorizes that the toxins may interfere with the transport of progesterone and possibly other hormones into the various cells of the body. Hormones can do their job only if they are transported to normal cells via the bloodstream. If progesterone fails to reach its destination the result might be PMS.

Candida produces more than toxins; it also produces hormones that are similar to estrogen and several metabolic by-products. A normal number of Candida organisms do not produce enough hormones to create an imbalance, but large numbers of Candida naturally secrete large numbers of estrogen-like hormones, which then affect the balance between estrogen and progesterone. Dr. Remington explains, "Candida by-products can also interfere with the ability of cells to receive estrogen, in a sense 'competing' with the estrogen. Other by-products can compete with the body's hormone actions in many ways, which may explain the irregular menstrual periods, infertility, and miscarriages suffered by many candidiasis patients." An overgrowth of Candida may also draw hormones away from the cells that need the hormones. The Candida organism is not only capable of absorbing hormones, but even has receptor sites specifically for steroid hormones on its cell walls.

Men

Although Candida overgrowth is more commonly associated with women's health problems, men are also affected. Men have a similar but slightly different set of symptoms from women. Dr. Crook writes that typical male patients "tend to be tired, irritable, and depressed. They're often plagued by recurrent headaches and digestive disorders, and their work productivity is reduced. Moreover they may be troubled by prostatitis and a diminished sex drive."

In his essay "Chronic Candidiasis and Allergy," George F. Kroker, M.D., lists the symptoms frequently reported by adult males (his list is similar to one by Dr. Crook). Dr. Kroker lists fatigue, depression, bowel disturbances, low-grade irritability, chronic prostatitis, allergies, and carbohydrate and yeast cravings as being typical Candida-related symptoms among males. Often the history of an adult male includes chronic infections, chronic fungal skin infections, use of multiple series of antibiotics, use of steroids for allergies, and sexual partners with yeast infections.

Dr. Truss stresses that the medical history of each patient is crucial to a correct diagnosis: "When this behavior pattern develops, especially if associated with intestinal symptoms, acne, and a history of allergy, infections, and antibiotics, yeast infection and allergy should be considered. It is only one of the possible causes of this type problem, but again, the consequences when this diagnosis is missed are tragic."

Dr. Truss notes that since men lack progesterone, their symptoms tend to surface in the form of chronic fatigue and a bad disposition, instead of the wide range of emotional symptoms seen in women. It is partially because men lack these emotional symptoms that Candida-related problems in men are often hard to diagnose. Dr. Truss writes, "As a result, this condition in men is less easily recognized; its constancy gives the impression that this is the normal character and personality. Missing are the clues to the diagnosis furnished by women by menstrual abnormalities, the resurgence of vaginitis, and abrupt mood swings, all frequently traceable to the use of an antibiotic or birth control pills, or to repeated pregnancies, etc."

The list of symptoms below is specifically for men and varies somewhat from the general problems that arise from Candida. Men should suspect yeast problems if any of the following are true:

- They have food and inhalant allergies.

- They have recurrent fungal infections like "jock itch," athlete's foot, or fungal infections of the nails.

- They have taken broad-spectrum antibiotics repeatedly for acne, prostatitis, sinus problems, or infections.
- They have consumed large quantities of beer, bread, and sweets, and they crave alcohol.
- They have other family members who are bothered with Candida-related problems.
- They have symptoms of unwellness on damp days or feel ill when exposed to chemicals, car exhaust, or tobacco.
- They have sexual problems such as a diminished sex drive or impotence.
- They have peculiar nervous system disorders such as fatigue, depression, or irritability.
- They have recurrent digestive system problems such as constipation, diarrhea, and abdominal pain.

Even if men don't appear to have a problem with Candida, they may need treatment if their wives or sexual partners have a Candida-related illness.

The effects of Candida overgrowth in men aren't usually as devastating as they are for women, according to Drs. John Parks Trowbridge and Morton Walker. They believe this is because women's more complex hormonal system may set them up for trouble. "Furthermore, men suffer less frequently from candidiasis, probably because they are not generally treated by doctors as often as are women, so they are exposed less often to the wonders—and resulting difficulties—associated with modern medical technology," write Drs. Trowbridge and Walker.

"Men can be just as sick as women, but for men it is harder for Candida to get out of control," said Dr. Truss. Men lack progesterone, which affects women from puberty until menopause. Men also have different anatomical structures and are less likely to have the urinary tract infections or cystitis that encourage antibiotics to be prescribed as treatment. "And finally, in contrast to men, sexual intercourse tends to aggravate the yeast problem in women. Yeast growth is rare on the male genitalia; significant growth in men is restricted to the intestinal tract and possibly the prostate gland," writes Dr. Truss.

Although men do have fewer problems with Candida, the results can still be shattering. "Although for reasons given, this condition appears to be less common and less easily recognizable in the male, it can have equally devastating effects on intellectual performance and mood, and can be equally destructive of self-confidence and accomplishment," emphasizes Dr. Truss.

Children

Children are frequently exposed to two of the factors that cause Candida growth: antibiotics and diets high in sugar and yeast. Children are often given antibiotics for recurring ear infections, which are common among young children and infants. Pediatricians and family physicians prescribe over $500 million worth of antibiotics each year alone for childhood ear infections. Another $500 million is spent on antibiotics to treat other childhood illnesses. As an alternative to prolonged antibiotic therapy, nystatin, which does not promote Candida growth or weaken the immune system, can be successfully used.

Doctors at the University of Southern California recently made a discovery that further supports research on the negative affects of antibiotics and Candida growth. They found that excessive doses of antibiotics used to treat ear infections in children contributed to the growth of yeast in the middle ear. An antifungal drug, ketoconazole (Nizerol), successfully treated the growth. Two studies have also shown that children who receive antibiotics for middle ear infections are almost three times more likely to have recurrent ear infections than children who receive a placebo. The reason may be that children are able to develop their own natural immunity to infections, but that antibiotics interfere with this natural response.

Diagnosing Candida-Related Problems in Children

Figuring out whether or not a child has Candida-related problems is very different from diagnosing an adult patient. The basis for an adult diagnosis is usually reliance on a medical history that shows known contributors to Candida growth, such as the use of antibiotics or birth control pills. A diagnosis is also frequently based on the symptoms that characterize CRC.

Doctors should look for some of the same things, however, when making a diagnosis of Candida-related problems in children as they do when examining adults. Dr. Remington lists three predisposing factors that may indicate Candida infection. The first factor is superficial Candida infections a child may have as a baby, such as thrush or diaper rash. He adds that although these problems do eventually go away, they may indicate the tendency toward future problems. The second predisposing factor is poor nutrition, whether from a lack of appetite or from foods that lack nutritional value. The third is heavy or even casual use of antibiotics. Dr. Remington writes that although frequent antibiotic use is most often the culprit, even occasional antibiotic use can cause candidiasis. He adds that if your child has one of the predisposing circumstances and at least two of the following symptoms usual in children with CRC, Candida-related problems are "highly probable." Another possible sign of Candida infection may be if he or she continues to be bothered by frequent infections.

The common symptoms of Candida-related problems in young children can be broken down into six general categories: gastrointestinal problems, behavioral and learning problems, musculoskeletal problems, emotional and mental problems, sugar cravings, and allergies. Gastrointestinal symptoms include abdominal pains or stomach aches, cramps, gas, bloating, and frequent diarrhea. Behavioral and learning problems encompass difficulties such as poor memory, learning disabilities, hyperactivity, attention deficit disorder, unusual aggressiveness, autism, or other noticeably inappropriate behaviors. Since hyperactivity and autism are behavioral problems a number of parents are forced to deal with, more information on them is included later in this chapter.

Musculoskeletal symptoms range from overall muscle problems such as aches and cramps to fatigue and poor muscle coordination. Emotional and mental problems can manifest as depression, irritability, intense anger, frustration, and rapid mood swings. Sugar cravings are fairly self-explanatory, and allergies include everything from asthma, hives, eczema, and the various symptoms of allergic reactions and food, inhalant, and chemical sensitivity. Dr. Remington notes that allergies that begin after the use of antibiotics particularly point to a Candida infection.

In infants the symptoms are a bit different. In his essay Dr. Kroker lists the prevalent symptoms of Candida-related problems in infants as carbohydrate cravings, hyperactivity, irritability, and chronic bowel disturbances. The typical history of an infant with Candida may include frequent use of antibiotics, chronic infections, and yeast infections. Prior diagnoses may have included the statement that the baby is "failing to thrive." Upon examination, oral thrush, diaper rash, and the common signs of allergy may be present.

Early diagnosis of Candida illnesses cannot only help you avoid other related problems in the future, but can even help you strengthen your immune system. Many patients who learn of their Candida problems during adulthood also report common Candida-related symptoms in their childhood, like frequent diarrhea and constipation. Allergies are another warning flag that should not go unheeded. As Dr. Truss points out, allergies can and do have serious consequences: "It must be reiterated that other allergies can have similar effects on brain function, as can nutritional deficiencies, toxic substances, and undoubtedly other physical factors of which we are yet unaware."

Dr. Truss describes a situation that sometimes occurs in infants after prolonged use (usually seven to ten days) of a potent antibiotic: "Restlessness, discontent, and irritability often accompany the 'runny nose' [a clear nasal discharge not previously present] and are responsible for the infant's inability to sleep restfully or without interruption for the normal duration." Dr. Truss further cautions that nasal discharge can lead to further infections since the inflamed mucous membrane cannot resist other germs.

Teenage girls are at risk for developing Candida-related problems for two reasons: once they reach puberty, progesterone begins circulating through their bodies, and if they are prone to acne, they may be given antibiotics, most commonly tetracycline. Teenage boys with Candida-related problems may be depressed, ill-tempered, lack ambition, and have severe acne. "School work suffers severely as a result of the intellectual impairment, the lethargy, and the depression; school drop outs are frequent among both boys and girls with this problem. (After seeing a number of these cases one cannot help wondering about the possible relation of this condition to the sharp increase in teenage suicide and drug use)," writes Dr. Truss.

Several steps can be taken to prevent Candida infections in children, which may then prevent potential problems in adulthood. Four suggestions to help parents stop problems before they start are to use antibiotics sparingly, and when they are used to accompany them with Lactobacillus supplements; to breast-feed infants; to completely treat thrush, a common childhood complaint; and to avoid refined carbohydrates and artificial sweeteners as much as possible.

Antibiotics should be used only when a definite bacterial infection is present, and broad-spectrum antibiotics should be avoided whenever possible. Penicillin, specifically penicillin V or penicillin G, or Erythromycin are generally effective without killing good bacteria. Lactobacillus should be used at the same time and for two weeks afterward. If Candida-related problems usually develop after antibiotics are used, nystatin should be used at the same time as the antibiotic and for two weeks after the antibiotic is discontinued.

Breast-feeding not only helps prevent general infections by providing a certain amount of immunity, but may also guard against Candida infections as well. Breast milk contains special Lactobacillus organisms and chemicals that help promote the growth of other good organisms. Commercial baby formulas and regular cow's milk lack Lactobacillus. Many infant formulas also contain refined carbohydrates, often from corn, which may feed the Candida organism.

Too often the treatment of thrush is incomplete or inadequate. Although thrush is known to indicate a decreased immune response, it isn't always taken as seriously as it should be. The standard treatment is Mycostatin oral suspension. Unfortunately, this medication contains 50 percent sugar, which is known to contribute to Candida growth. And although the manufacturer recommends that Mycostatin be continued for forty-eight hours after the thrush has disappeared, this may not be long enough to eliminate the excess Candida in the intestinal tract. The usual recommended dosage of two hundred thousand units four times a day probably is not enough to get rid of excess Candida either. This treatment of thrush also ignores the importance of restoring the normal balance of Lactobacillus bacteria in the body.

Eliminating refined carbohydrates (including sugar) and artificial sweeteners from your child's diet is another way to prevent Candida-related problems. Proper nutrition keeps the immune system running, which helps fight off infection and chronic illness.

Hyperactivity and Autism

Hyperactivity and autism are behavioral problems that are frequently associated with children and may be connected to Candida. While there is no evidence to assume the two health conditions have anything to do with each other, there is reason to believe they may be connected to the toxins emitted by Candida.

Both Dr. Truss and Dr. Crook suspect that Candida plays a role in some childhood health problems, including hyperactivity and autism. This reasoning makes sense given that sugar and other food allergies have been linked to both CRC and hyperactivity. Antibiotics may also influence or trigger hyperactive behavior. Dr. Crook reports that treating hyperactive children with an anti-Candida therapy, which includes dietary changes and nystatin, produces significant results: "Now that I've become aware of Candida-related illness, I feel some hyperactive children, especially those who have taken repeated courses of antibiotics, react to sugar because the sugar triggers Candida." Based upon his clinical experiences, Dr. Crook has changed the way he treats many illnesses, including ear infections, behavioral and learning problems, and hyperactivity.

As mentioned earlier, the toxins emitted by Candida are what cause the myriad symptoms associated with CRC and what stimulate allergic reactions. These toxins can affect all of the organs of the body, including the central nervous system. Disturbed brain function is thought to play a part in depression, anxiety, and memory problems and may play a big part in more serious autoimmune diseases and mental illnesses such as schizophrenia and manic-depressive psychosis. These toxins are especially suspected in the case of autism because many doctors report that autism has responded favorably to anti-Candida treatment.

What distinguishes hyperactivity from normal childhood behavior is *excessive* movement and restlessness. Symptoms associated with and often present with hyperactivity include: being "spaced out" or inattentive, an inability to concentrate, irritability, mood swings, overactivity, aggressiveness, hostility, learning problems, short attention span, fatigue, depression, headaches, ear infections, bed-wetting, digestive problems, muscle and joint pain, constant infections and colds, and allergies.

Autism is a serious disturbance of mental and emotional behavioral growth. It is characterized by the extreme versions of these behaviors: abnormal withdrawing into oneself, inability to interact socially, severe communication problems, short attention span, and resistance to change. Autistic children can also be extremely difficult to teach. The causes of this abnormal behavior are still unknown, but since many physicians have successfully treated autism with a Candida-control diet and therapy, the cause may be linked to Candida.

Both autism and hyperactivity have responded favorably to what is called an "elimination diet," a diet very similar to the one recommended for CRC patients. This type of diet involves eliminating foods that may cause allergic reactions in children. Dr. Crook recommends that parents initially eliminate sugar, milk, wheat, chocolate, corn, soft drinks, sugary drinks like Kool-Aid and punch, eggs, food colors and dyes, and processed and packaged foods. Recent articles and research suggest food additives and foods can alter the normal function of the body, especially the nervous system.

Dr. Crook, who started practicing pediatrics in 1949, ran a bustling general pediatric practice during the 1950s and 1960s. He has noted that incidents of hyperactivity and autism and other behavioral problems have been rising during the last several decades.

Dr. Crook bases his list of foods on a study he conducted from January 1, 1973, through December 31, 1977. During this time Dr. Crook saw 182 new patients with hyperactivity and attention deficit problems and seven new patients with autistic problems. Of the 182 hyperactive patients, 136 responded to dietary changes; their parents noticed a definite improvement in their children's behavior. The foods found to cause the most symptoms were the ones listed earlier to initially eliminate from your child's diet. Dr. Crook also put the autistic patients on a special diet that helped eliminate foods they were allergic to.

One example of an autistic child who responded to treatment is

Ann. After age one, she exhibited autistic symptoms such as regressed speech and being spaced out. After the child was put on the special diet, Ann's mother listed the allergic food reactions she observed in her: sugar caused moodiness, irritability, and disagreeable personality; corn, wheat, and other grains led to hyperactivity, hallucinations, bizarre facial expressions and gestures; and milk caused her to be irritable or to space out. Although the diet alleviated many of the symptoms, an orthomolecular psychiatrist discovered considerably high levels of lead in Ann's hair, blood, and urine. The levels were decreased through prescription megavitamins.

Other physicians have also successfully treated hyperactive children by controlling their diets. A great deal of research has been done on the possible effects of foods and food additives to attention deficit hyperactive disorder (ADHD). This is a common problem that affects between 3 and 10 percent of the population. Not only can it be frustrating for parents, it can also stunt children's emotional and social growth. What causes this problem is presently unknown, but the fact that children improve dramatically when their food allergies are determined and the offending foods are then eliminated from their diets is encouraging.

A definitive article on ADHD in children was written by Marvin Boris, M.D., and Francine S. Mandel, Ph.D., and published in May 1994 in the *Annals of Allergy*. The article stated that diet plays a "significant" role in the cause or origin of ADHD in a majority of children. The foods that were held suspect included dairy products, wheat, corn, soy, citrus fruits, yeast, eggs, chocolate, and peanuts. Artificial colors and preservatives were also eliminated. A full 73 percent (nineteen of the twenty-six children) showed improvement after these things were eliminated from their diets for two weeks.

Over the next month, the children were challenged with one suspicious food item every two days, and each child who reacted was given the same food item again. The researchers then offered each child his or her particular allergenic food item hidden in another food that masked its smell, flavor, and texture. Children received a placebo or a challenge item at random. Allergenic responses were found in 69 percent, or eighteen of the children.

Of the nineteen children who showed improvement as a result of the elimination diet, seventeen were found to have allergies. Of the seven children who did not improve, five did not have allergies. A significant difference in hyperactivity was found between the placebo and challenge days. The researchers found that "the difference of behavior between the children's original diet and the elimination diet was substantial." Based on their findings, Drs. Boris and Mandel recommend that symptoms can be controlled through a simple elimination diet and that challenge tests after a broad elimination diet can aid in determining which foods are responsible for the hyperactive behavior. They also conclude that, "Elimination of the causes of ADHD is preferable to the pharmacologic therapy of this condition."

Candida-related problems are extremely serious in children. They can interfere with children's normal growth and development, disrupt their performance in school, and make them prone to develop allergies and cycles of infections. Childhood is the foundation upon which adult health is based, and poor health in these early years can have far-reaching consequences.

—5—

What Causes Candida Growth?

It seems, indeed, a necessary weakness of our minds to be able to reach truth only across a multitude of errors and obstacles.
—Claude Bernard in *An Introduction to the Study of Experimental Medicine*

Half of what we have taught you is wrong. Unfortunately, we do not know what half.
—Dean Burwell, M.D., to Harvard medical students in *The President's Report*, 1982-83

Identifying what causes Candida growth is important for two reasons. It helps us recognize which circumstances can lead to CRC and lets us know which changes to make in our lives to avoid or treat it.

Stress: Candida's Best Friend

As previously mentioned, what causes Candida-related illness is not exactly the Candida organism itself, but what allows it to grow out of control. And one of the largest contributors to its overgrowth is a compromised or weakened immune system. What causes the immune system to fail to function properly can be summed up in one word: stress.

Stress comes in many forms and can have a tremendous effect on our health. It can be interpersonal, occupational, environmental, nutritional, emotional, or physical. We are perhaps most familiar with emotional stress—our individual and often negative reactions to what happens in our lives. But the stress that assaults our health includes much more than just anxiety or tension.

The most common forms of stress are biological, environmental, emotional, deprivational, social, and familial. Biological stresses include microorganisms from inside and outside us that can decrease the effectiveness of our immune system such as bacteria, viruses, yeast, parasites, fungi, and mold. Environmental stresses are conditions and factors surrounding us such as noise, extremes of temperature and humidity, lack or excess of sunlight, air or water pollution, or traumatic accidents. In small quantities, environmental stresses may not be very damaging, but when one factor or several factors combine together, the result can be overwhelming. Anger, hostility, cynicism, resentment, anxiety, hatred, fear, and other negative emotions define emotional stress. Deprivational stress means having enjoyable emotions and events withheld from us, such as humor, laughter, joy, love, fun, sleep, and exercise. Social stresses involve events that may not always personally involve us, but still affect us in some way, such as crime, racism, war, and other world events. And finally, familial stresses include divorce, marriage, death, birth, separation, changes in financial or work status, abusive relationships, and any other changes which may create stress.

Recognizing the potential stresses around you is important, but research shows that it is also crucial to learn how to deal or respond to stress. How each of us views potential stress factors and our abilities to cope with them are vital to the influence stress has on our lives.

Stress has physiological effects on the body and is linked to immune system function. It starts a chain reaction throughout the body, starting with the brain, which sends a message to the hypothalamus, which in turn stimulates the pituitary gland, which then stimulates the adrenal cortex to release corticosteroids. Corticosteroids, which are listed later in this chapter as a type of drug that increases Candida growth, are chemical compounds that regulate the immune, cardiovascular, and other systems. They are also frequently prescribed to reduce inflammations such as rheumatoid arthritis. One of the known side effects of corticosteroids is increased susceptibility to infection and, when an individual is under prolonged stress, corticosteroids can suppress the immune system.

Stressful situations, in particular illnesses and stressful life events, have been linked to several diseases including diabetes mellitus, cirrhosis of the liver, heart disease, and asthma. Stress is suspected in contributing or causing other illnesses, according to Eve Potts and Marion Morra, authors of *Understanding Your Immune System*:

Studies show a much wider range of disorders associated with the experience of stressful events. There are illnesses in which the mechanism by which stress could cause disease is less obvious but which clearly involve the immune system in some way. They range from colds to influenza, from tuberculosis to arthritis and cancer, from lower back pain to recurrent flare-ups of herpes, skin blemishes, and allergies.

The link between stress and infection was first noticed around the turn of the century by Tohru Ishegami, M.D., an infectious disease specialist. Dr. Ishegami was studying patients with tuberculosis (TB) and found stress predicted who would become sick with TB and who would not. He found "The principal factor determining whether tuberculosis patients would survive or succumb to this infectious disease was their emotional state," write Drs. Michael A. Schmidt, Lendon H. Smith, and Keith W. Sehnert in *Beyond Antibiotics: 50 (or so) ways to Boost Immunity and Avoid Antibiotics.* Dr. Ishegami found that TB patients had similar personal histories that had in common various failures and other distressful events, such as unsuccessful businesses or unhappy family lives. He also noticed that nervous individuals were more likely to have attacks of TB and that people with chronic cases of TB would improve until some unfortunate incident occurred. Then their health would decline.

Although Dr. Ishegami's ideas were published in 1919, it wasn't until 1980 that there was an effort to understand the connection between infection and stress. It took more than sixty years for this idea to be rediscovered, and only in the 1990s has it been fully recognized and confirmed by research. Drs. Schmidt, Smith, and Sehnert note: "This 'novel' concept that stress and life events might influence the course of infectious disease was published in 1919. Since Dr. Ishegami's time, the germ theory of disease and antibiotic treatments dominated the medical scene. Little attention was given to the psychosocial aspects of infection."

Although no one will say stress causes infections, research has shown that there is an association between stressful life events and illness. One study by Drs. R. J. Meyer and R. J. Haggerty, published in *Pediatrics* in 1962, followed sixteen families for one year. Each member of each family had a physical exam that included a throat culture for streptococcal bacteria every three weeks. Each member also kept a diary to track events throughout the year. At the end of the year researchers made these conclusions: stress was four times more likely to come before an infection than to come after an infection; when throat cultures showed streptococcal bacteria to be present, 50 percent of those under high stress became ill; conversely, of the low-stress family members with positive strep cultures, only 20 percent became ill; and finally, 25 percent of the outbreaks of illness followed a family crisis.

Since there is evidence to support a link between immune system function and stress, those suffering from Candida-related illnesses should pay close attention to how they manage the stresses in their lives. One of the most important sources of stress to our immune systems is the misuse of antibiotics.

Antibiotics and Your Body

Along with an impaired immune system, antibiotics play one of the biggest roles in triggering CRC. Many physicians consider broad-spectrum antibiotics, a type that kills a wide range of organisms, to be the most frequent contributor to it. They contribute to Candida growth in two ways: by killing the bacteria inside us that normally help regulate Candida growth and by weakening our immune systems.

Not all bacteria in our bodies are harmful; many of them actually serve a positive role in our health. One obvious example is the bacteria that keep Candida under control. Without that bacteria, Candida can grow unbridled and cause problems throughout the body. Marc Lappé, Ph.D., author of *When Antibiotics Fail: Restoring the Ecology of the Body*, reports that there is overwhelming evidence that many bacteria naturally protect us. Several species of bacteria on the skin, for instance, protect against pyoderma, impetigo, strep throat, and *Staphylococcus aureus,* which is a major cause of skin infections. Other bacteria boost the immune system by stimulating defense mechanisms and encouraging the body to produce antibodies that neutralize foreign substances, including the Candida organism and its toxins.

Antibiotics, especially broad-spectrum antibiotics, kill more than the microorganisms they are prescribed to get rid of; they also wipe out these helpful bacteria. Indirectly, they can even encourage the growth of harmful types of bacteria by creating a noncompetitive environment for them. Stuart Levy, M.D., a longtime crusader for careful antibiotics use and author of *The Antibiotics Paradox*, compares the situation to a lawn overgrown with weeds. "Once the ecosystem has been cleared of bacteria, resistant bacteria can multiply or enter into the noncompetitive arena. The phenomenon can be likened to weeds that have overgrown a lawn where the grass has been completely destroyed by an overdose of herbicides." Dr. Levy is a professor of medicine and microbiology at Tufts University School of Medicine in Medford, Massachusetts.

Antibiotics also interfere with our natural immunity. Mildred S. Seelig, M.D., author of an article on the mechanisms by which antibiotics increase the incidence and severity of Candida infection, is one of many authors who links antibiotics use to decreased immunity. Dr. Seelig writes: "Production of antibodies to *C. albicans* in normal subjects provides evidence both of symptomless tissue invasion and of building up of defenses. Evidence has been presented that broad-spectrum antibiotics inhibit antibody synthesis, and that tetracyclines [a type of antibiotic] depress the levels of the globulin fractions that have been shown to possess *Candida*-cidal activity." Dr. Seelig later asserts that antibiotics have been shown to hinder both antibody synthesis and phagocytic activity, the engulfing of foreign particles by the cells of the immune system. The end result is reduced host resistance to Candida invasion.

How much antibiotic use is too much can depend on many factors including the dosage, the type of antibiotic, and the immune system of the person taking the antibiotic. High doses of antibiotics may be damaging to your body, as can repeatedly switching from one antibiotic to another. Long-term use (daily use for several months), such as the daily use of tetracycline to control acne, can also be too much.

A Legacy of Misuse

Every day a sniffling, sneezing patient walks into a doctor's office, and if a viral infection is suspected, antibiotics are prescribed. The scenario is repeated over and over again in America even though antibiotics are useless against viruses, the organisms that cause colds and flu. Going to the doctor to get antibiotics has unfortunately become almost routine. But it is important that patients realize the detrimental effects it can have on their health. Overuse of antibiotics also lessens the effectiveness of medicine in healing as germs become drug resistant through overexposure to them.

Antibiotics are frequently given by doctors as a quick fix to an uncertain problem. Sometimes there is little investigation by the doctors to determine the real problem. And after prescribing an antibiotic, he or she may give scant medical advice on how to take it correctly. The best way to diagnose and treat an infection is to take a culture, and after examining the results, prescribe an antibiotic that would kill that specific bacteria. Dr. Lappé cites a recent study at twenty different hospitals. It found that over one-third of the antibiotic treatments were begun without "a culture being performed to determine the sensitivity of the strains involved to the antibiotic used." When cultures were performed, the researchers found that 39 percent of the patients who would have been given antibiotics did not receive them, as it was unnecessary.

Unfortunately the realities of general medical practice today make culturing every infection unrealistic and impractical. Physicians don't have quick access to labs, and they can't delay treating ill patients who are frantic to get well. Faced with an unknown enemy and the knowledge that many bacteria are now drug resistant, doctors may prescribe a broad-spectrum antibiotic that is more powerful than regular antibiotics and that will kill more types of bacteria (unfortunately, both helpful and harmful). This frequently suits the hurried patients, who want no more disruption in their lives than taking a pill three times a day.

Patients also bear some responsibility for the overuse of antibiotics. Unaware of the repercussions, they may demand antibiotics from their doctors or even shop around for someone who will prescribe antibiotics on demand. Many patients do not finish their prescribed course of antibiotics, thus contributing to the overall problems with antibiotics by enabling some bacteria to survive and become drug resistant. Antibiotics also help bacteria to become drug resistant when they are used too frequently. Patients are unaware of how to best use antibiotics, and doctors don't think to provide that information.

Doctors also prescribe antibiotics for prophylactic, or preventative reasons, in an effort to discourage possible infections. Often doctors believe they can bridge a gap in times of insufficient immune response in this way. The beliefs behind prophylactic use of antibiotics are not illogical or inconsistent with good medical practice, but prophylactic use doesn't always work, nor has it been widely studied or tested by the medical community. Too often doctors do it not with the patient's welfare in mind, but rather to minimize possible future legal problems for themselves. Dr. Lappé writes, "In an age of litigation, some surgeons tend to use prophylactic treatment as part of the practice of defensive medicine."

Not only is the long-term health of the patient at stake, but also the overall health of the community. To protect their patients from overmedication Dr. Lappé advises physicians to tailor the treatment to the needs of the patient instead of doing what is convenient for themselves:

> Physicians are going to have to recognize that the best possible treatment for the patient may not always be the best possible treatment for the hospital, the community, or the

next generation of patients to come. "Blitzing" a seriously
ill patient with broad-spectrum antibiotics to get that extra
bit of insurance that an infection is controlled represents
neither good medical practice nor sound clinical judgment
if the long-term need for health protection of the community is factored in.

There are certain instances when prophylactic use of antibiotics
is warranted and even necessary. Some physicians and surgeons
agree that antibiotics should be given before open-heart surgery
and surgery of the gastrointestinal tract due to the high risk of possible infection. Other surgical procedures in which prophylactic
antibiotics may be useful in *possibly* helping to sterilize the blood
and intestinal tract are hysterectomies, high-risk cesarean sections,
colorectal surgery, total hip replacement, and head and neck
surgery. However, an article in *Modern Medicine* shows that 70.9
percent of antibiotics used prophylactically in the hopes of preventing postoperative surgery were "irrational on the basis of
proved efficacy" and only 7.6 percent of antibiotics prescribed after
postoperative surgery were used in what the researchers described
as a rational manner.

Although antibiotics are frequently used by physicians to reduce
the risk of infection in the cases of serious viral respiratory infections, burns, chronic disease, or trauma, research shows they may
actually be ineffective. Research conducted by leading experts in the
field say time and time again that antibiotics have been proven not
to prevent infection when used in these cases.

Because of these misconceptions and simple carelessness, the
problems that cause disease go unsolved and get worse. In their book
*Candida Albicans: How to Fight an Exploding Epidemic of Yeast-Related
Diseases*, Ray C. Wunderlich, M.D., and Dwight K. Kalita, Ph.D.,
emphasize that an illness doesn't occur because a single germ is present and we happen to be exposed to it. They write:

> It is essential to understand, therefore, that in the real
> world infectious illness occurs not because some "germ"
> arbitrarily decides to attack our bodies. Rather, illness
> occurs because our nutritionally deficient, debilitated bod-
> ies permit these microbes to set up residence. In short, an
> opportunist microbe is an infectious agent that produces
> disease only when the circumstances are favorable.

Whether or not you develop an illness or disease depends not on
exposure to germs, but on your individual immune system defenses.
If your immune defenses are tired or worn out they cannot protect
against microbial infection.

Antibiotics: A Daily Part of Our Lives

Despite the growing problems associated with antibiotics, their use is increasing. Sales have doubled since the 1980s and have risen steadily in the past several years from $3.7 billion in 1988 to $5.6 billion in 1993. Obstetricians and gynecologists write more than 2.6 million antibiotic prescriptions every week, and internists write 1.4 million per week. Antibiotics account for 10 percent of all prescription drug sales. The rise in the use of antibiotics is understandable given the announcement in 1994 by *The New England Journal of Medicine* that during the 1990s there has been a worldwide explosion of bacterial and viral diseases.

Another reason for the increase in sales is that so many bacteria are becoming drug resistant, so antibiotic after antibiotic has to be tried, adding between $100 million to $200 million each year to America's health-care bill. Antibiotics consume 40 to 50 percent of the pharmaceutical slice of hospital budgets. Some U.S. hospitals spend one-quarter of their budget alone on vancomycin, a new and highly powerful antibiotic that, as use grows, is also becoming less and less effective.

Studies conducted in the past several decades have reached an ominous conclusion: 50 to 60 percent of all outpatient prescriptions are inappropriate and seven in ten people with common colds (which are caused by viruses) receive antibiotics even though antibiotics cannot kill viruses. Our difficulties with antibiotics are a symptom of a larger problem: overuse of both over-the-counter and prescription drugs is a regular part of many Americans' lives. By seeing drugs as unquestionable cure-alls and by overusing them, we have created additional medical problems for ourselves.

Taking prescription antibiotics is not the only way to become exposed to them. We often ingest them along with things we eat. Many of us don't realize the extent to which antibiotics are present in our food or that for most or all of our lives we have all been exposed to long-term low levels of antibiotics.

Antibiotics are introduced into the food chain through farm animals, specifically turkeys, chicken, pigs, and cattle. Farm animals are given antibiotics to enhance growth and prevent the spread of disease. In fact, farm animals actually receive thirty times more antibiotics than people do. Most of these drugs are forms of penicillin and tetracyclines. Animals receive antibiotics directly and also consume them in their food. According to the U.S. General Accounting Office (GAO), 143 drugs (including antibiotics) and pesticides are likely to leave residue in raw meat.

Much of the milk we pour on our cereal every morning contains minute amounts of eighty different antibiotics. Farmers use these antibiotics on their cows to prevent udder infections (mastitis).

Although the United States Food and Drug Administration (USFDA) sets restrictions on the amounts of antibiotics that can be present in milk, we may all be exposed to higher levels than anyone realizes. A 1992 study by the General Accounting Office (GAO) found that states test for only four of the eighty allowed antibiotics. In addition, the GAO's own tests detected trace amounts of sixty-four antibiotics at levels they said "raise health concerns."

Antibiotics, when used correctly, are extremely beneficial to humankind. As Dr. Levy writes, "Antibiotics are a medical treasure, perhaps the most important therapeutic discovery in the history of medicine. But they are being misused." Like most treasures, it is important not to take them for granted or we will all end up paying the price.

Antibiotics and CRC

Many of the physicians who treat CRC agree on at least one thing: although many factors encourage chronic problems with Candida, antibiotics use is the number one contributor. A brief list of the antibiotics that can encourage yeast growth includes amoxicillin, ampicillin, Bactrim, Ceclor, Erythromycin, tetracycline, Keflex, and penicillin.

As mentioned previously, the overuse of antibiotics promotes problems with Candida in two known ways. The first is that broad-spectrum antibiotics, which are used to kill *some* bacteria, actually kill *a wide variety* of bacteria, many of which normally function to keep the Candida organism from growing out of control. The second way is that antibiotics can inhibit some of the normal defensive mechanisms of the immune system.

One important beneficial bacteria is *Lactobacillus acidophilus,* which lives in the mouth, intestinal tract, and vagina and which is also found in cultured milk products, specifically yogurt. *Lactobacillus acidophilus,* also called acidophilus, helps in the digestion of food and the manufacture of folic acid and vitamins B_1, B_2, B_3, and B_{12}. In the early days of antibiotics, from about 1950 through 1965, physicians were advised to routinely give patients *Lactobacillus acidophilus* to compensate for the amount of good bacteria antibiotics killed. The first such product was Lactinex. Adding *Lactobacillus acidophilus* capsules or tablets to the diet is one way people with Candida can restore the disturbed ecology of their bodies. When shopping for Lactobacillus supplements, make sure the product has been refrigerated and contains only one strain.

We each have about four hundred different species of microorganisms inside or on us. They all compete for space in our intestinal system, on our skin, and in general throughout our bodies. The result of this normal competition is a balanced relationship. As Dr. Remington writes, normally the microscopic organisms establish a balanced relationship with each other and with the host (you) by competing for their space.

In *Beyond Antibiotics: 50 (or so) Ways to Boost Immunity and Avoid Antibiotics* Dr. Sehnert talks about his experiences with antibiotics and urges patients to explore options other than antibiotics and to improve their immune systems and nutritional status. Dr. Sehnert recently conducted a survey of three thousand patients he treated for CRC to find out what had caused their problems. Over 90 percent reported that before their illness started they had "excessive and prolonged" use of broad-spectrum antibiotics. Leo Galland, M.D., a physician who has treated hundreds of patients with Candida-related problems, reached the same conclusions about antibiotics and CRC. Dr. Galland studied ninety-one patients with CRC and found that antibiotics were a precipitating factor in 82 percent of the patients.

Dr. Baker agrees with the importance antibiotics play in the onset of CRC. He refers to the topic as "tipping the balance." About antibiotics Dr. Baker writes, "The quickest way to get some sort of yeast problem is to take a lot of antibiotics. Within days after doing so, many people may experience symptoms related to a change in the flora of our intestine, mouth, or vagina." In addition to taking acidophilus supplements, another way to prevent or help stop Candida overgrowth from antibiotics is to also take an antifungal drug such as nystatin while taking the antibiotic.

In her 1966 article in the *American Journal of Medicine,* pioneer Dr. Seelig states clearly that antibiotics have increased Candida infection. She writes: "Investigators have proved that antibiotics, by suppressing the growth of the usual flora, permit the outgrowth of antibacterial-resistant species. Antibacterial therapy, particularly with broad-spectrum antibiotics, and/or mixtures of antibacterials, thus encourages overgrowth of fungi, the most common of which is *C. albicans.*" Dr. Lappé also cautions against overuse of antibiotics and makes a point of mentioning Candida overgrowth when summing up the dangers of overuse of antibiotics. He describes what happens to the ecology of the gut when antibiotics are introduced:

> Once "cleared" of harmful and helpful bacteria alike, parts of our bodies became the aforementioned wastelands where only the most opportunistic organisms could gain a foothold and proliferate. Sometimes now, as with vaginal "yeast" infections, this overgrowth begins as a simple irritation. But in many people, the proliferation of

yeast cells called Candida albicans runs amok, spreading system-wide disease.

Before repeating that antibiotics increase Candida growth, Dr. Lappé hints at the growing awareness toward CRC in the medical community. He then goes on to say,

> Some specialists in the new medical discipline of clinical ecology believe that Candida may be responsible for a wide range of diseases including asthma, depression, diarrhea, and even autism. While the jury is still out on these last attributions, there is no doubt that antibiotics encourage the overgrowth of Candida and other undesirable pathogens.

Further medical texts and articles also support the link between antibiotics and Candida growth.

There is no question that antibiotics have been and will be extremely beneficial to humankind. It is how we choose to use them that is the problem. Several difficulties have resulted from overuse of antibiotics, with two prominent ones being the overgrowth of Candida in the body and drug-resistant bacteria. While in some respects the evolution of drug-resistant bacteria was inevitable and anticipated by the medical community, the problems with Candida are not only unexpected but also unnecessary.

Medications other than antibiotics can increase Candida growth. Prescription steroids and corticosteroids are good examples. They affect Candida growth by disrupting the normal protective inflammation in the body. Steroids are frequently prescribed by doctors to suppress inflammation and to treat arthritis, asthma, and allergies. Corticosteroids are steroids produced by the adrenal cortex or are prescription drugs that produce an effect similar to the steroid from the adrenal cortex. Frequently prescribed steroids are cortisone and prednisone, both commonly used to treat inflammations. Prednisone is also used to treat rheumatoid arthritis, sinusitis, and allergic reactions. Steroids also shut down the body's defensive mechanisms and weaken the immune system. Other side effects include increased susceptibility to infection and emotional changes.

Diet and Your Body

Nutrition plays a big part in how we feel and function. Diets that contain foods with little nutritional value, especially sugar and junk food, increase Candida growth in our bodies. Foods that contain simple carbohydrates also increase Candida growth and should be avoided.

Nutrition and Infection

Poor nutrition and infection are closely connected. Inadequate nutrition impairs the normal function of the immune system, making it easier for organisms to come in and establish themselves in our bodies. Once we are ill, nutritional deficiencies hinder recovery, and illness itself further depletes nutrients from the body, weakening our defenses even more. Infection can cause the body to use up stored nutrients, such as vitamins C and A and zinc. Doctors have known for a long time that rheumatoid arthritis, acute tonsillitis, pneumonia, measles, and even fevers reduce the amount of vitamin A in the body, which then makes patients more receptive to further bouts of illness. It makes sense, then, that proper nutrition not only aids our recovery from illness, but also helps us fight off infection to begin with.

Nutrition and Candida Infection

Research done by Leo Galland, M.D., and published in *The Journal of Orthomolecular Psychiatry*, shows that nutritional deficiencies accompany Candida infection with high frequency. Dr. Galland lists magnesium, essential fatty acids, and vitamin B_6 as being standard deficiencies after instances of invasive Candida infection, such as vaginitis. "Deficiencies of each of the three nutrients have been demonstrated to suppress immune function," he writes. Besides having a general immunodepressant effect, magnesium deficiency also impairs antifungal defenses. Magnesium deficiency is associated with several medical conditions long associated with CRC, including allergies, PMS, and mitral-valve prolapse.

Magnesium, essential fatty acids, and vitamin B_6 are extremely important in maintaining health. Magnesium plays a crucial role in proper enzyme activity, and deficiencies cause nervousness and irritability. Essential fatty acids are the building blocks of lipids (energy reserves), and since they are not manufactured by the body, they must be obtained through diet. Vitamin B_6 affects both physical and mental health and is involved in more bodily functions than any other nutrient. Vitamin B_6 is also required for normal function of the brain and nervous system.

Dr. Galland performed metabolic studies on 104 patients seen during a one-year period. All of the patients had Candida allergies or toxicity and all met criteria similar to the definition of CRC. In addition to the nutrient deficiencies list above, he also found low stores of iron, depressed serum folate, and low levels of vitamin A. Dr. Galland also noted that since iron deficiencies have been shown to predispose one to Candida infection, low levels in patients with Candida infections should be taken seriously.

According to Dr. Galland, other researchers have found that magnesium deficiencies are widespread in the United States and that both essential fatty acids and vitamin B_6 are missing from American bodies in epidemic proportions. He reports that since the three nutrients work together, a deficiency of one might engender deficiencies of the other two. Dr. Galland believes that the deficiencies start when patients begin taking antibiotics. He observed:

> Many Candida patients seem to develop their nutritional problems after exposure to antibiotics. Some [patients] behave like Mg sieves, requiring 1000-2000 mg of Mg a day to avoid deficiency. Nutritional therapy alone is merely palliative in most patients, and specific antifungal therapy is required for optimum therapeutic response.

Like antibiotics, nutritional deficiencies weaken immune defenses and predispose a host to Candida infection. The Candida organism takes advantage of this favorable situation and multiplies, often causing CRC. As Dr. Galland states, "The success of *C. albicans* as a modern parasite may lie in its ability to further undermine our weakest metabolic links."

A 1991 article in the *Journal of Surgical Research* supports the theories about Dr. Rhinehart's findings concerning nutrition and the body's ability to perform metabolic functions. The article clearly states that "protein-calorie malnutrition (PCM) is recognized as the most common cause of immunosuppression worldwide." This article specifically studied how protein-calorie malnutrition impairs the host's defenses against *Candida albicans*. Although the authors never actually define PCM, they do say it is common in underdeveloped countries and in developed countries among the elderly, hospitalized patients, and some small infants. Their results, however, can be applied beyond malnourished patients. The authors declare: "Our results demonstrate the importance of nutritional status in maintaining host defense mechanisms against fungal invasion. Moderate malnutrition was associated with greater gut mucosal invasion by *C. albicans*, higher organ colonization, and delayed organ clearance." Clearly poor nutrition not only weakens the body, but also prevents it from naturally cleansing itself of harmful substances.

Sugar and Other Junk Foods: Big Problems in Tasty Packages

Of all the foods that can damage the body, sugar seems to be the most effective. Sugar is sweet but has no nutritional value, lowers immune defenses, and encourages Candida growth. Having the occasional treat will probably not damage the body. However, if large amounts of sugar are consumed on a daily basis, the result may be an immune system unable to fight infection.

"Limiting the intake of sweets and starches deprives Candida of the nutrient that allows its maximum multiplication," writes Dr. Truss. Dr. Crook sums up the relationship between sugar and yeast growth: "Feeding sugar and simple carbohydrates to Candida organisms is like pouring kerosene on a fire."

Dr. Lorenzani describes sugar as the "twentieth century food." Given that the average American consumes more than 130 pounds of sugar every year—fourteen times more than was consumed only one hundred years ago—this statement rings true. Obvious evidence of our need for sugar is everywhere, especially in shopping malls and supermarkets. Many supermarkets dedicate entire aisles to cookies, candy, syrups, sugar-coated cereals, and ice cream treats and desserts. Less obvious examples of sugar-laden foods are tucked throughout the store: some examples are beverages, like fruit juices and soda, that contain large amounts of sugar.

Some foods that are less apparent sources of sugar include condiments like ketchup and mustard, salad dressings, fruit juices, dried fruits, and fresh fruits. Molasses, maple syrup, and honey are also forms of concentrated sugar. Even most toothpastes contain refined sugar or a concentrated chemical form of sugar. An average day in the local shopping mall shows people flocking to the many cookie, ice cream, and candy stores—all thriving businesses.

Sugar is not just a part of our diet, but also our lives. Holidays are remembered and celebrated by the candies that define them. Christmas wouldn't be Christmas without candy canes and gingerbread houses. Giving heart-shaped chocolate candy to a loved one is part of the ritual of Valentine's Day and is equivalent to saying "I love you." Easter hops into town preceded by solid chocolate rabbits with yellow or pink bow ties and jelly beans in every color of the rainbow. And the queen of all sugar-coated holidays is, of course, Halloween, when almost everyone buys candy in anticipation of trick-or-treaters.

Sugar has little nutritional value and provides only carbohydrates that are quickly used by the body. Sugar contains no A, B, C, D, and E vitamins and no minerals whatsoever, two elements essential for human life. In fact, sugar has so little nutritional value it is often referred to by nutritionists as a "dead food."

Several studies comment on the effect sugar has on the body. One concerns sugar's effect on the white blood cells that fight infections by eating invaders. One type of white blood cell that is affected by sugar is neutrophils. Not only do neutrophils fight infections, they also consume tissue debris, aiding the body in repairing damaged tissue. Dr. Lorenzani writes:

Neutrophils do their best work when blood sugar levels are neither too high or too low. In other words, homeostasis [the normal state of equilibrium in the body] helps white blood cells do their job. When blood sugar climbs too high or drops too low, as it often does after the consumption of sugar, honey or even orange juice and apple juice, neutrophils appear almost paralyzed. It is then that infectious organisms can have a heyday.

Sugar basically deadens the blood cells that protect us against infection. A report published in the *American Journal of Clinical Nutrition* found that one hundred grams of sugar from sucrose, glucose, fructose, honey, or even orange juice caused a significant decrease in the ability of white blood cells to perform their main purpose, which is to destroy foreign substances in our bodies. This decrease in function lasted five hours.

In addition to weakening the immune defenses that protect us against Candida infection, sugar also feeds the Candida organism. Candida thrives on simple carbohydrates like the ones found in a wide variety of sugars, including cane and beet sugar, honey, molasses, and corn and maple syrup. Eating fruits also promotes Candida growth because fruits, which are high in fructose, are converted to simple sugars in the body. Some low-sugar fruits are not as harmful.

White flour is another example of a food product that can encourage yeast growth. It can easily be broken down into simpler carbohydrates that feed Candida. (Milk also contains large amounts of simple carbohydrates, and it is a good idea to avoid both of these foods.) In addition to providing Candida with nutrients to grow, refined flour is also lacking in many of the nutrients essential to proper immune function. Although it isn't surprising that refining the whole wheat grain into white flour decreases the nutrients, the actual percentages of lost nutrients paints a scary picture. The refining process results in drastic nutritional losses:

- 89 percent less cobalt
- 86 percent less manganese
- 85 percent less magnesium
- 78 percent less zinc
- 68 percent less copper
- 48 percent less molybdenum
- 40 percent less chromium

These aren't the only nutrients lost. Other casualties include selenium, essential fatty acids, and vitamin E. What does stay in the flour is cadmium, a harmful heavy metal that would have been countered by the zinc if it hadn't been removed. In order to get the required nutrients from your food, try to eat whole-grain products whenever possible.

Like sugar, junk foods lack nutritional value and put additional stress on the immune system. Junk foods are refined, processed, and full of hidden ingredients. They are also loaded with sugar, salt, food coloring, additives, chemicals, and hardened vegetable oil. Some examples are soft drinks, processed snacks, and fast foods.

Leftovers can be unhealthy because they are more likely to contain yeasts and molds. In addition, nutrients naturally decrease as time passes, so leftover foods often contain few nutrients. Chemical processes and additives also lower the nutrient value of food. Preservatives, coloring agents, foaming agents, binders, thickeners, stabilizers, and emulsifiers also remove valuable nutrients from food.

People with CRC should avoid sugar and junk food whenever possible. Make sure you read every label and select restaurants carefully; even French fries are frequently deep fried with sugar to promote browning.

Food Allergies: An Often Undiagnosed Contributor to Illness

It is important for those with CRC to consider the possibility of food allergies for multiple reasons. First of all, food allergies can alter immunity, further exacerbating CRC. In addition, the leaky gut problem common to CRC sufferers can contribute to food allergies, making CRC patients more susceptible to them. James C. Breneman, M.D., former chairperson of the Food Allergy Committee of the American College of Allergists, estimates 60 percent of the population has unknown or hidden food allergies. Only about 5 percent are aware of their allergies, which leaves 95 percent unaware of the role some foods play in their health and wellness. Recent research suggests foods and food additives have the ability to alter the normal function of the nervous system.

An allergy is an individual's sensitivity to a substance that in similar amounts does not provoke a response in other people. An allergic reaction is basically a false alarm caused by the immune system when it mistakenly attacks a harmless substance. "The immune system cannot distinguish between dangerous intruders such as bacteria or parasites and innocent ones such as grass pollen or house dust, or even beneficial ones such as milk and eggs. If the material is perceived as foreign, the immune system goes on to attack," write Eve Potts and Marion Morra, authors of *Understanding Your Immune System*. The symptoms characterized by an allergic reaction, which often include sneezing, wheezing, runny nose, and irritated eyes, happen because of a chemical substance released inside our bodies by our immune system when the offending substance is present.

While the terms *food allergy* and *food intolerance* are often used interchangeably, such usage is incorrect. An allergy specifically involves an abnormal response from the immune system, while an *intolerance* or *sensitivity* is a broader term that applies to any unpleasant and nonpsychologically based reaction to a specific food or food ingredient.

Allergists consider a *true* food allergy one that provokes an elevated level of certain antibodies in the blood. One common example is the easily recognizable symptoms, which include a facial rash, some people experience after eating strawberries.

Incidences of allergic reactions seem to be increasing, and the reason may be our increasing exposure to chemicals in our food, environment, and increasingly potent medications. As Drs. Schmidt, Smith, and Sehnert write in *Beyond Antibiotics*, "Many doctors note that this type of reaction is growing in frequency as we consume more processed foods, are exposed to more chemicals, and use more antibiotics."

Two illnesses previously thought to have been caused by bacterial infection have been shown to be linked to food intolerances. A recent study published in *Family Practice News* and presented at the 1991 meeting of the American College of Allergy and Immunology by T. M. Nsouli, M.D., showed that of 104 children with chronic middle ear infections, 78 percent (eighty-one children) tested positive for negative reactions to foods. After the foods they tested negatively for were eliminated from their diets for eleven weeks, seventy of the eighty-one children improved noticeably. When the offending foods were again reintroduced into their diets to confirm the suspected food allergies, sixty-six of the eighty-one children again developed middle ear infections.

Tonsillitis is another illness linked to food intolerance. A recent article in the *Journal of the Royal Society of Medicine* says that cow's milk is one of the major causes of chronic tonsillitis. Other illnesses that are suspected to be caused or aggravated by food intolerances are respiratory tract infections (associated with food or airborne allergies), bladder infections, and sinus infections.

"Allergy doesn't cause everything, but it can cause anything," declares an old clinical observation. Both clinical experience and research have shown this statement to be true. And because we are all different and have different needs and reactions, any food can cause an allergic reaction. In children, the foods responsible for 80 percent of adverse reactions are cow's milk, peanuts, eggs, and soy products. In adults, the list of most common offenders is similar but longer and includes dairy products, including butter, milk, cheese, cottage cheese, ice cream, and yogurt; anything that contains wheat, including bread, cereal, gravies, cookies, and crackers; peanuts or other nuts; and citrus fruits and juices, especially oranges. Other offenders are all forms of chocolate, soy, eggs, corn, shellfish, sugar, and yeast.

While milk is popularly believed to be one of the healthiest substances available, research these days tells us this is not always the case. Milk does provide calcium, which is necessary for strong teeth and bones, but it has been connected to recurrent ear infections in children. Many patients, usually children, who need tubes placed in their ears are sent to Fred Pullen, M.D., an ear, nose, and throat specialist in Miami, Florida. Dr. Pullen first put these patients on a diet that completely eliminated dairy products and found that 75 percent of his patients did not need to have tubes implanted in their eardrums.

What Causes Food Allergies?

According to J. O. Hunter, M.D., "Food allergy is one of the most controversial topics in medicine." Dr. Hunter is the author of a hypothesis on what may cause food allergies, which was published in 1991 in *The Lancet*. The idea that foods can lead to illness has been greeted skeptically by the medical community.

Many factors are suspected in causing or leading to food allergies and intolerances, including the leaky gut problem discussed in chapter 3. Drs. Schmidt, Smith, and Sehnert present many possibilities, including a genetic tendency toward allergies and using large amounts of antacids, aspirin, or ibuprofen (or other anti-inflammatory drugs), which thin the intestinal lining and prevent proper absorption of nutrients. Antibiotics are another culprit because they can also thin the intestinal lining and prevent absorption of nutrients. According to Drs. Schmidt, Smith, and Sehnert, this can lead to the development of intolerances of foods. When the helpful, normal bacteria inside us have been decreased, often from antibiotics use or by drinking heavily chlorinated tap water, the possibility of food intolerances increase.

Dr. Hunter proposes two possible causes of food allergies. The first is reduced enzyme concentrations in the body. People who have low levels of liver enzymes, which are necessary for the complete breakdown of food, may have food residues pass into their circulation as a result. These residues are seen as enemies by the body, which attacks them and causes the allergic reactions. Dr. Hunter also agrees with Drs. Schmidt, Smith, and Sehnert that disrupted flora in the bowel may contribute to food problems. If food allergy is found not to be an immunological problem but rather one based on disrupted bowel flora, the entire definition of food allergy would change. According to Dr. Hunter: "This is of more than mere terminological importance: modern microbiology has opened the way to the manipulation of bacteria flora to allow the correction of food intolerances and thus the control of disease."

Poor nutrition also contributes to food intolerance. "Consumption of the wrong types of fats, too much sugar, too much junk food, too little fiber, too few vegetables, and too little fruit makes it difficult for the absorption of nutrients to take place properly. It also makes it difficult to build new cells that line the digestive tract," write Drs. Schmidt, Smith, and Sehnert.

Another possibility might be intestinal infection by viruses, parasites, or bacteria. In one study of patients affected with *Giardia lamblia*, a common parasite found in contaminated water and food throughout the world, a full 100 percent were intolerant to lactose, the sugar found in milk. "Doctors have known for years that viral infection of the intestine results in temporary intolerance to food. For example, children who suffer diarrhea due to the common rotavirus suffer from food intolerance that lasts several weeks," write Drs. Schmidt, Smith, and Sehnert.

Food allergies and intolerances can be determined by looking at three areas: medical history, symptoms, and allergy tests. If you have a history of allergies, especially in childhood, or if your family has a history of allergies, then you may have food allergies. One reason food allergies can be so hard to detect is they cause both immediate (type 1) and delayed (type 2) reactions. The delay period between eating the food and the negative reaction can be hours or even days.

There are four standard food allergy patterns: fixed, cumulative, variable, and additive. A fixed reaction is the type of reaction that happens every time you eat a certain food. Cumulative reactions take place after a certain amount of food has been eaten either immediately or over the period of a couple of days. One amount may not provoke a reaction while another amount may. An example is a child who may not have a reaction after one glass of milk at dinnertime but may feel ill after two or three glasses of milk. Variable reactions are unpredictable and fail to follow a rational pattern. Examples are women who react to a certain food only during their menstrual cycles or children who can sometimes tolerate chocolate and sometimes not. And finally, addictive reactions describe the withdrawal symptoms that people often associate with certain foods. Common withdrawal symptoms include headaches, irritability, cravings for the addictive food, depression, anxiety, weakness, shaking, and fatigue. When the addictive food is eaten, the symptoms disappear. Dr. Remington writes, "Many of our patients who have given up addictive food have noticed the clearing of troublesome symptoms that plagued them for many years. In most cases they had no idea that ingesting these foods on a daily basis was causing these problems." Dr. Remington also notes that a food allergy/addiction situation is impossible to win: you feel poor if you eat the addictive food and even worse when you don't eat it. The only rational solution is to completely eliminate the food from your diet.

The common symptoms of food allergy fall into four basic areas: respiratory symptoms such as sinus, nasal, or bronchial congestion, frequent colds and earaches, and coughing; intestinal symptoms such as bloating, cramps, loss of appetite, gas, nausea, constipation, or diarrhea; skin problems such as hives, eczema, patches of dry skin, or seemingly unexplainable rashes; and general emotional or physical symptoms such as irritability, fatigue, headaches, depression, tension, or insomnia. Changes or problems that affect the eyes are another characteristic of food allergies and include wrinkles under the eyes, puffy eyes, or bags under the eyes.

Testing for allergies is done three different ways: blood tests, skin tests, or food-elimination tests. Although allergists frequently use scratch tests of the skin to determine allergies, most recognize that scratch tests do not always detect food allergies or intolerances, or sometimes inhalant allergies. A more reliable skin test called the intradermal cutaneous test involves injecting a small amount of the suspected substance beneath the skin and then waiting for a possible reaction.

Several types of blood tests are available. One test is called the ELISA/ACT test and is available from Serammune Physician's Lab in Reston, Virginia, and Immunolabs of Ft. Lauderdale, Florida. This test has been closely examined by researchers and found to be accurate in determining delayed-type or late-phase allergic reactions, which are the types frequently missed by older allergy tests. This test is also helpful in determining sensitivity to the environment and various foods. The IgG antibody test measures reactivity to a wide variety of substances, including environmental allergens (such as molds, dust, and mites), airborne allergens (such as pollen), environmental chemicals, foods, food additives, and preservatives. The third type of test is the food-elimination test, which involves eliminating foods known to commonly cause allergic reactions. The foods are avoided for one to four weeks. Suspicious foods are added one at a time, and if an allergic reaction results, the suspicious food is then considered to be the cause and permanently eliminated from the diet. "Elimination-provocation is still considered the 'gold standard' among allergy tests. Its main limitation is that it requires time, effort and compliance on the part of the patient," write Drs. Schmidt, Smith, and Sehnert.

Just as antibiotics and nutritional deficiencies place stress on the body, so can food allergies and intolerances. If you suspect that allergies are part of your problem, talk to your doctor about what allergy tests are available and what he or she may recommend. Finding any previously undetected allergies will take stress off an already overloaded immune system and improve your overall health.

Birth Control Pills and Hormonal Fluctuations

Hormonal changes or fluctuations promote the growth and multiplication of Candida in the body. Hormones are chemicals that regulate the activities of groups of cells or organs. Two hormones that affect sexual characteristics in women are progesterone and estrogen. For women, hormonal changes occur during adolescence, the normal menstrual cycles, and pregnancy. Birth control pills, which contain synthetic versions of progesterone and estrogen, also cause hormonal fluctuations that favor overgrowth of Candida.

Oral contraceptives, approved by the FDA for contraceptive purposes in 1960, suppress fertility in women by preventing ovulation, the release of an egg from the ovary. Birth control pills are also commonly used to control menstrual irregularities and are generally considered safe for women under age thirty-five.

Birth control pills have long been recognized as a frequent contributor to CRC. Physicians and scientists who have studied this problem all list birth control pills as encouraging yeast growth and as part of the medical history that may signify CRC. When discussing treatment of CRC, Dr. Truss emphasizes the importance of avoiding birth control pills and explains the part they play:

> Rivaling antibiotics in impact on the immune containment of Candida have been the "birth-control pills," whether used for contraception, prevention of menstrual cramps, or regulation of menstrual irregularity. Avoidance of these hormones is mandatory if chronic candidiasis is to be successfully controlled. Chronic yeast vaginitis tends to be at its worst when progesterone levels are high, as in pregnancy and the luteal phase of the menstrual cycle; therefore the progesterone component of contraceptive hormones may well be responsible for their adverse effect.

Birth control pills encourage Candida growth because progesterone causes changes in the mucous membranes of the body, which in turn affect the Candida organisms living in the membranes. Drs. Trowbridge and Walker speculate that, given the evidence available, birth control pills help "meet the metabolic needs" of the Candida organism. "Oral contraceptives probably promote Candida colony growth through a direct and unavoidable mechanism," write Drs. Trowbridge and Walker.

Dr. Crook also recognizes the role birth control pills can play in increasing Candida growth. He writes:

> The progesterone component of these pills causes changes in the vaginal mucous membrane, which makes it easier for ever-present yeasts to multiply and cause not only vaginitis, but associated systemic symptoms, including irritability, fatigue, and depression. Other mechanisms may be involved in producing these symptoms, including changes in hormonal function.

According to Dr. Lorenzani, the progesterone content of the pill creates the perfect vaginal environment for Candida to multiply. She also ties progesterone in with increased vaginal inflammation: "It has also been observed that nonpregnant, nonpill users with chronic yeast infections have a flare-up of symptoms during the two weeks prior to their period. This coincides with the stepped up progesterone released between ovulation and the monthly period." Dr. Lorenzani also points out that an estimated 35 percent of women on the pill have severe yeast vaginitis, a fact that further supports the link between progesterone and Candida overgrowth since vaginitis is a common symptom of CRC. Dr. Truss also came to the same conclusions about birth control pills, noting that: "Their use is associated with acute vaginal candidiasis in approximately 35 percent of women."

Chemicals: Another Stress on Our Bodies

Some people report that chemicals such as pesticides have brought on Candida-related problems and that they have allergic reactions to the chemicals around them. The Human Ecology Action League (HEAL) recognizes chemical sensitivities and environmental illnesses. It is a nonprofit volunteer organization that has chapters throughout the U.S.

HEAL reports that people vary greatly in their response to chemicals and that some have no reaction or a very mild reaction while others, who are more vulnerable, become very ill. HEAL lists the most vulnerable as women, the young, the elderly, the poor, allergy sufferers, the chronically ill, and workers in high-risk occupations who are exposed to chemicals frequently. One reason these groups may be vulnerable is because their immune systems may be weaker. Unborn and young children may not have fully developed immune systems, and any of the groups listed earlier (especially the poor and the elderly) may not eat properly and therefore may be nutritionally deficient.

Your Toxic Load

The phrase *toxic* or *chemical load* has gained popularity over the past few years in describing the cumulative effect chemicals from our home and environment can have on our bodies. Basically the term *toxic load* describes the total number of apparent or latent chemicals affecting your health.

Exposure to chemicals can be gradual and in limited doses, or all at once, such as exposure to insecticides or to weed killer. Small amounts can have an additive effect on our bodies and over time greatly weaken our immune defenses. We may not even be aware of the chemicals around us. "Exposure to low amounts of formaldehyde in the home, gasoline from the garage, nitrogen oxides from the smog downtown, lead in the drinking water, colorings in the food, prescription drugs, etc., all add up to what's known as the total toxic load. Individually, these substances may be present in such small amounts as to be insignificant. Collectively they add up to a heavy burden," write Drs. Schmidt, Smith, and Sehnert.

A 1994 article in *Newsweek* magazine discusses growing awareness of a new finding: repeated exposure to a common chemical substance can lead to severe and even life-threatening allergic reactions. The substance is latex rubber, which is used to make condoms, surgical gloves, balloons, and hundreds of other products. Because the latex used to make condoms is highly purified, condoms are less likely than other latex products to cause allergic reactions.

Allergies to latex appear to be more common than first suspected and are now deemed a significant public-health issue. Two high-risk groups are health-care workers and children who undergo numerous operations. A Milwaukee immunologist estimated that 10 to 17 percent of all health-care workers are allergic to latex, and 30 to 60 percent of all children who have undergone numerous operations are also allergic to latex. Although these high numbers are not surprising given these two groups are at a higher risk than other people, recent investigation has shown that 6.5 percent of the population at large is at least partially sensitized to latex rubber.

These findings are significant because they give hope that other chemical sensitivities will now be recognized by mainstream medicine and perhaps solutions will be found. Latex problems have been recognized by both the FDA and the American College of Allergy and Immunology, and in 1992 both issued warnings about latex. Given the research on latex and the fact that exposure to this chemical substance has such obviously negative effects, there is reason to believe the long-term harmful effects of other chemical substances on the body will also be given the research and attention the matter deserves.

According to Dr. Crook four variables determine how sensitive each one of us is to the chemicals around us and whether or not we will become ill. They are our inherited tendencies; the total load of chemicals we are each exposed to every day (in our food or in the environment around us); the amount of other allergic problems around us, such as pollen, mold, and foods; and the strength of our immune systems.

Like CRC, signs of a toxic body do not fit into neat categories. The symptoms that characterize a toxic body are also similar to the most prominent CRC symptoms. Drs. Schmidt, Smith, and Sehnert describe the symptoms this way: "In general, symptoms of toxicity are very vague and broad. Fatigue, sluggishness, and just a low level of wellness are hallmarks." Normally reported symptoms can be separated into two categories: mental/cognitive and physical. The mental symptoms include lethargy, fatigue, depression, nervousness, and irritability. The physical symptoms are chronic infections, allergies, frequent colds, sluggishness, chemical sensitivities, reactions to strong odors, headaches, and muscle and joint aches.

When we become overloaded with toxins our immune systems become lazy and slow. If we are challenged by an infectious organism, including Candida, the immune system cannot adequately respond and an infection results.

Chemicals and Our Bodies

Recent research done by Joseph Beasley, M.D., and published in *The Kellogg Report* in 1989 describes how exposure to chemicals can leach the nutrients essential for growth and renewal out of our bodies. Three nutrients especially crucial to the immune system are the vitamins A and C and the mineral zinc. A few of Dr. Beasley's findings follow: workers who were exposed to pesticides suffered from a severe disruption in their levels of vitamin A; being subjected to even small amounts of PCBs (an environmental pollutant that can accumulate in animal tissues) decreases the levels of vitamin A stored in the liver of animals by half; more than twenty cigarettes per day decreased blood levels of vitamin C by 40 percent; and insufficient vitamin E worsens the effects of nitrogen dioxide from smog, a mixture of fog polluted with smoke.

HEAL recommends that people who experience suspicious symptoms should clean up their surroundings by determining and then reducing sources of indoor pollution. Common sources of indoor pollution are scented products, pesticides, household cleaners, tobacco smoke, gas appliances, heating and ventilating systems, office machines, and construction materials.

Dr. Crook advises patients to stay away from chemicals and details how they play a role in making people sick. He stresses: "If you suffer from a yeast-related illness, learn as much as you can about chemicals and how to avoid them." He points out the difference between helpful chemicals, which are part of our bodies, and foreign chemicals, which can hurt us. Some chemicals normally present in the body are salt, potassium, calcium, and magnesium. Foreign chemicals are often made from petroleum and other sources and can include fumes and fuels such as gasoline, natural gas, diesel fumes, garage fumes, coal-burning stoves, and wax candles. Walk through your home and workplace and observe everything around you that is made of chemicals. Products and objects made of synthetic materials have become a part of daily lives and may be contributing to feelings of chronic unwellness.

Other ordinary products to avoid are cleaning fluids; nail polish; formaldehyde; brass, metal, or shoe polish; floor waxes; furniture polishes; clothing dyes; disinfectants; cosmetics; asphalt pavements; inks; and carbon paper. Objects made of rubbers, plastics, and synthetic textiles are also the sources of frequent chemical complaints. Sources of rubber include sponge rubber, foam rubber pillows, typewriter pads, rubber-based paints, and automobile accessories. Plastics include plastic upholstery, pillow covers, bags, handbags, food containers, dishes and utensils, kitchen appliances and cookware, phones, computers, doors, plastic cement, and tape. Synthetic textiles include dacron, polyester, and rayon.

Cosmetics, because of their chemical content, are also a frequent source of irritation. Some things to watch out for are soaps, hair shampoos, hair conditioners, deodorants, antiperspirants, hand lotions, antiseptic preparations, face powders, nail polish and nail polish removers, eye makeup, hair spray, antiseptics, perfumes, colognes, shaving lotions and creams, scented toilet paper, aftershave lotions, and douches.

Physical stress can come in many forms. To keep your immune system strong, your defenses up, and Candida growth regulated, there are several things you can do. Avoid emotional stress, antibiotics, a high-sugar diet, birth control pills, and chemicals in your environment whenever possible.

—6—

You and Your Doctor

The doctor is not primarily a scientist. He (or she) is a person who has been trained to think, to observe critically, and to realize that a human being is not a conglomeration of integrated complex systems, but an individual with a personality of his own.
—William A. R. Thomson in *Institute of Public Health and Hygiene*

In *The Missing Diagnosis*, the first book to break the silence about yeast-related illnesses, C. Orian Truss, M.D., discusses the role of yeast in human illness and assures readers that this illness is not the fault of patients, nor is it psychosomatic. Published in 1983, *The Missing Diagnosis* was the first American book to put a name on this chronic illness that affects many people whose problems have been downplayed by their doctors. Dr. Truss, an internist and allergist in Birmingham, Alabama, writes: "For many men and women, this diagnosis has been the answer to their collective plea to doctors to find the cause of their chronic symptoms and to 'please stop trying to hang this on us.'"

Much research still needs to be done before we can fully understand CRC, but fortunately that is not the main concern of a growing number of physicians. Although proving and disproving theories and determining exactly how CRC affects our bodies is important, it is more important to find effective treatments and help sick people regain their health. There are many things scientists and physicians don't understand about the human body. For example, no one knows what triggers labor in a pregnant woman. Although we may never know, this certainly doesn't stop us from having children or from working around that missing piece of knowledge. Fortunately today, doctors are beginning to take that approach in regard to CRC.

Finding the right doctor can make the difference between recovering from your illness in one year and recovering in two years or more. In fact, it can determine whether or not you even get a correct diagnosis of your problems. The information in this chapter emphasizes the need for you to work closely with and communicate with both your partners in this venture: your physician and your pharmacist. The goal of this chapter is to give you the information you need to make the medical decisions in your life and to effectively communicate your needs and problems. (For specific advice on physicians and medications, consult chapter 11.)

Getting a Correct Diagnosis

Getting an accurate diagnosis is crucial to recovery because your doctor will base decisions about your care on it, including what medications you will need to take and for how long. The treatments for CRC are rather specific, and a doctor who suspects you have a stomach flu isn't likely to recommend them to you. Further, an incorrect diagnosis could lead to treatments (such as a course of antibiotics) that actually exacerbate your problems.

The majority of physicians follow three procedures before determining that Candida is the source of a particular patient's health problems. The three steps include a thorough examination of the patient's medical history, an analysis of his or her symptoms, and a laboratory test of either a blood or stool sample or both. If the patient recovers after several months of diet and antifungal therapy, then the diagnosis is confirmed.

One of the best ways for a doctor to measure your symptoms and determine your medical history is through the use of a questionnaire.

Questionnaires: A Guide to Symptoms and Medical History

One common tool used by doctors to diagnose Candida-related illnesses is a health questionnaire. A doctor may write her own or use one provided by one of the authors of books on Candida-related illnesses. One regularly used questionnaire explores a patient's medical history as well as his or her major and occasional symptoms. One of the more important questions asks what medications the patient has taken, since both antibiotics and birth control pills are known to affect Candida growth. Based upon the answers to the many questions, a score is determined. Although a diagnosis can be predicted based on the score alone, many doctors may also want to order lab tests. The diagnosis is either confirmed or denied based on a positive or negative response to the anti-Candida therapy, which usually involves diet modifications and antifungal medications.

Questionnaires, which are also called symptom scoring systems, are used to diagnose a number of medical conditions that lack laboratory tests. Some examples of illnesses or medical conditions in which questionnaires are frequently used include mental illnesses such as depression and anxiety. Questionnaires are also used to diagnose and measure stress and to predict the probability of survival of cancer patients. Rheumatic fever, an infectious disease, is diagnosed based on symptoms. The Centers for Disease Control (CDC), the governmental agency responsible for the investigation, diagnosis, and control of disease in the United States, developed a questionnaire in 1988 to determine the diagnosis of Chronic Fatigue Syndrome (CFS).

Dr. Crook stresses the need for a physicians help in getting a diagnosis and says that getting a correct one "takes a suspicion by a physician." Although questionnaires are extremely helpful in diagnosing CRC, they cannot replace a careful examination of your medical history by your doctor. As Dr. Lorenzani writes in *Candida: A Twentieth Century Disease*, "Diagnosis of Candida is not a do-it-yourself project. An experienced physician is invaluable in diagnosing and guiding one through the recovery process."

A Wide Range of Symptoms

As described in chapter 2, patients with CRC can exhibit a wide range of symptoms. The symptoms are sometimes so diverse, in fact, that it is difficult to keep track of them all. This complexity of symptoms coupled with the many factors of health and lifestyle that may predispose a patient to CRC, can make diagnosis a cumbersome task. In *The Yeast Syndrome*, John Parks Trowbridge, M.D., and Morton Walker, D.P.M., try to simplify the process somewhat by dividing Candida-related symptoms and details of a patient's history that may signify CRC into seven broad categories:

- Frequently reporting a wide variety of apparently unexplainable symptoms.
- Having taken broad-spectrum antibiotics.
- Having taken birth control pills or having been pregnant.
- Having taken cortisone or other steroid medications.
- Having allergy problems or chemical sensitivities (negative reactions to everyday chemical substances).
- Having negative reactions to molds, fungi, or yeasts.
- Having unexplainable cravings for sweets, alcohol, or breads.

In addition to paying close attention to the factors presented in these basic categories, many doctors who treat Candida-related illnesses also stress the need for patients to listen to their own bodies. "Your present feelings and observations about yourself are every bit as valuable as any laboratory or physical examination," write Drs. Trowbridge and Walker. "Your physician will want to know what you sense about your own body's functions and how your mind and emotions are working."

Although there are a wide variety of possible symptoms, there are common threads that run through all of the diagnoses. Several of the most commonly reported symptoms, which happen to be mental/cognitive symptoms, are fatigue, depression, anxiety, irritability, and a feeling of unrealness also described as being spaced out. The common elements in a patient's medical history that, when paired with frequently reported CRC symptoms, generally indicate CRC are the use of antibiotics, especially broad-spectrum antibiotics; the use of birth control pills; a high-sugar diet; and the use of other immunosuppressant drugs, such as corticosteroid medications. The general consensus among doctors who treat this condition is that the overall medical history of the patient is the most important mechanism in reaching a correct diagnosis.

Your Medical History: An Important Diagnostic Key

Your medical history is important for several reasons. First and foremost, your history can help determine whether or not Candida is the cause of your health problems. Assuming your doctor does discover you have CRC, your medical history can point to when the problems started and what aspects of your health or environment caused them. Knowing what caused the problems lets both patient and physician know what behaviors to avoid in the future.

Doctors who treat Candida list the patient's medical history as the most significant indicator of Candida-related problems. Dr. Truss emphasizes that the "single most valuable diagnostic tool we have is an accurate medical history. This consists of symptoms and how they developed, of events to which they were related, and of factors that aggravate or relieve them. No detail related to symptoms should be omitted from the history, no matter how irrelevant it may seem to you."

There are certain fundamental points a doctor should consider when questioning you about your medical history to help him determine whether or not you have CRC. However, if your doctor isn't very familiar with Candida-related illnesses, he may not know what questions to ask. Remember these points listed in George F. Kroker, M.D.'s essay on Candida infection, and if your doctor doesn't ask you about them, volunteer the information on your own.

- What factors in your history might predispose you to excessive *Candida albicans* carriage?
- Is there any historical evidence of previous *Candida albicans* infections?
- Does there appear to be a correlation between increasing Candida antigenic load and increasing systemic symptoms?
- Is there a positive environmental history of food, mold, or chemical sensitivity?
- In taking the general medical history, are there any coexisting medical conditions that are usually associated with *Candida albicans* carriage?

An examination of your medical history, either orally or through a questionnaire, should also include the following:

- What medications you've taken, including antibiotics (especially broad-spectrum antibiotics,) birth control pills, steroids, cortisone-type medications (including skin creams), or other medications.
- Any past or present illnesses or medical problems you've had.
- Whether or not you've been pregnant.
- Whether or not exposure to strong chemical smells, such as tobacco, automobile exhaust, paints, or personal-care products makes you feel ill.
- Whether or not you crave foods made with yeast, alcoholic beverages, or sugar.
- Whether or not you've had any fungal infections, such as jock itch, athlete's foot, ringworm, or infections of the nails or skin.

Your medical history is a tool, and if you wish to get the most out of it, it must be accurate and correctly used. Before you visit your doctor, write out your medical history and symptoms based on the information listed above. Be careful not to leave anything out. By doing so, not only will you remember to tell your doctor all vital information, but you will also take your first step toward developing a partnership with your physician.

Diagnostic Tests for Candida

In his chapter on diagnosing CRC, Dr. Truss discusses the usefulness of established diagnostic tests, but acknowledges their limits: "This condition is first of all an infection; secondarily it is a response (allergic or toxic) to products of the infecting fungus that are reaching uninfected organs. Therefore the first effort in its diagnosis should be directed toward establishing the existence of an infection."

Dr. Truss explains the three types of tests used to detect infections: cultures, skin tests, and antibody levels. A culture is a deliberate growing of a microorganism in a solid or liquid environment. This is used to prove the microorganism is present in the site where the culture was performed. It also determines exactly how much is present. The other two types of tests, skin tests and antibody levels, indicate prior exposure to the microorganism but may fail to reveal whether that exposure is old or ongoing. And since we know Candida is present in both healthy and ill people, establishing that Candida is present doesn't do a great deal of good.

But despite their inadequacies, diagnostic tests are helpful to doctors. Even though they can fail to provide positive identification of a problem, they can sometimes reinforce a doctor's initial suspicions that Candida is the root of his patient's health woes. Although the tests can't positively determine a diagnosis, they can back up or throw doubt on a diagnosis suggested by the patient's medical history. "Fortunately the clinical picture is quite consistent, and in most cases the diagnosis can be tentatively made with considerable assurance. Earlier and milder cases require a higher index of suspicion, but usually respond more quickly to treatment so that the therapeutic trial is easier to apply," writes Dr. Truss. The treatment, which involves a revised diet and sometimes prescription medications, is a safe and effective medical approach toward yeast-related illnesses. No harm can be caused by trying it. Dr. Truss explains, "Treatment in such a situation is often termed 'a therapeutic trial'; the diagnosis is confirmed or rejected based on the response, or lack thereof, of the patient's symptoms and signs."

New Blood and Stool Tests for Candida

During the last decade blood and stool laboratory tests have been developed to test for CRC. In fact, blood tests for Candida overgrowth were developed more than ten years ago. If you wish to have a blood or stool test performed, consult your physician. If you don't have a physician, two labs that may be able to refer you to a physician in your area are Meridan Labs at (206) 631-8922 and Great Smokies Lab Client Services at (800) 522-4762.

Blood Tests

Blood tests measure whether or not the immune system has produced antibodies to fight Candida. The amount of antibodies present in the body can indicate whether or not the immune system is responding to an overgrowth of Candida, so blood tests are an ideal way to measure Candida overgrowth.

According to Aristo Vojdani, Ph.D., who is the vice president and owner of the Immunosciences Laboratory, Inc., in Los Angeles, if there is an overgrowth of Candida in the digestive system, it binds to the lining of the gut, which is called the mucosa. When Candida grows out of control in the digestive tract, Candida by-products enter the bloodstream and are carried throughout the body. The immune system views these by-products as foreign substances and produces antibodies to get rid of them.

Candida antibodies can be measured in a variety of ways. According to Dr. Kroker, opinions on the diagnostic values of yeast-antibody detection differ for three main reasons. One reason is that there is a lack of standardization of both testing techniques and antigen preparation. Secondly, antibodies to Candida commonly occur in normal human hosts who are free of disease, and finally, there is a "lack of established blood levels of *Candida* antibodies in disorders characterized by excessive *Candida* colonization." Despite these problems, serum tests are still useful indicators of Candida overgrowth.

Blood Tests: Insight into the Immune System

There are many labs around the country that use blood and/or stool samples to determine Candida infection. In blood tests only the serum, which is part of the fluid portion of the blood, is used. The serum is tested for the presence of three distinct Candida antibodies called "immunoglobulins," which are a class of structurally distinct antibodies produced in the lymph tissue in response to the invasion of an antigen, a foreign substance. The antibody molecule performs two different functions: antigen recognition and antigen destruction. The antigen in this instance is Candida. Even though it lives normally in the body, it is still a foreign organism.

Phillip Broughton, vice president of Antibody Assay Laboratories in Santa Ana, California, said that the measurement of antibodies alone is not a very good marker for active Candida overgrowth. One reason is that some types of antibodies produced by your body are present for only a brief time, though others remain for many years after the infection has subsided. This makes it difficult to tell whether you have a current Candida infection or whether you had one that has since gone away.

The serum test performed by Broughton's lab measures two things: the amounts of immunoglobulin antibodies and the patient's immune complex. His lab and other labs use a Candida-specific immune complex test to specifically measure Candida overgrowth. An immune complex is formed by the combination of antigens and antibodies. Tests have been designed to measure specific immune complexes. In the case of the Candida-specific immune complex, the test establishes the presence of an abnormally increased Candida load. Immune complex levels also drop quickly when the load is decreased, and this adds to the value of the test.

The immune complex test measures how the patient's body is clearing out the invading substance, in this case the Candida organism. As the amount of Candida increases the immune complex increases. According to Broughton, this close relationship between Candida and the immune complex is what makes it such a useful test.

Mary James, M.D., of Great Smokies Diagnostic Laboratory in Asheville, North Carolina, is in the educational services department and discusses patients' cases with physicians who use her lab. She also offers ideas on how each physician can tailor the necessary treatment for each patient. She receives about ten treatment calls a day (the simpler questions go to her lab's client services department, which she estimated may receive up to two hundred calls a day). She receives few calls concerning Candida tests, estimating that they comprise about 10 percent of the physician calls she receives.

When testing for Candida overgrowth, Great Smokies performs a test known as a comprehensive digestive stool analysis. Actually, this test is comprised of three different tests: the stool culture, the serum antibody, and a parasitology exam that measures for parasites. Dr. James describes the comprehensive test as being a "Candida intensive" test that measures a lot of other information as well.

Dr. James said that the comprehensive digestive stool analysis measures not just yeast and parasites, but also twelve other health variables. These measurements provide the physician with a wide range of information about the patient's overall health, including the condition of the mucosa and the gastrointestinal tract, which runs from the mouth to anus. Dr. James determines if the patient's sample shows an overgrowth of yeast, and then her lab tests for drug sensitivity and resistance. The lab then reports on which drugs or agents will be most effective against the Candida and gives guidelines for doctors to follow. Dr. James notes that a lot of samples show resistance to some of the drugs used against the yeast. She said drug-resistance testing is fairly standard practice among labs.

Jeff Beaman, a medical technologist at Great Smokies who has worked in the microbiology department for two years, said that not all of the yeast found in stools is *Candida albicans*; other varieties of the Candida family may also be present. Of the stool yeast cultures

Great Smokies performs, only about 50 percent or a little less are positive for yeast overgrowth, and about 80 percent of that yeast is *Candida albicans.*

Vojdani's Immunosciences lab also tests the immune complex as an indicator of Candida growth but uses a different measurement technique. The specialty of Immunosciences, which has been in business since 1988, is immunology. A total of six hundred doctors use the lab, with one hundred to two hundred doctors sending in Candida overgrowth samples from time to time. About 20 percent of the serum samples tested for Candida overgrowth indicate that it is present. The lab performs about two hundred such tests a month.

As a licensed lab in California, Immunosciences has to have a request from a licensed doctor to perform a test. As for payment, sometimes doctors pay for the test, sometimes patients send a check with the test, and sometimes Immunosciences bills the insurance company. By law doctors in California cannot charge more than the fee set by the lab, but laws on this topic differ around the country.

Each lab reported a turnaround time of about three to four days for antibody serum samples depending on the volume of testing at that particular time. Dr. James said the turnaround time for the stool culture is about a week, explaining that time is needed for the organisms to grow on the culture before being measured.

Laboratory Recommendations about Diagnosing Candida

Just as there are a wide variety of testing techniques for Candida overgrowth, there are also many different opinions and recommendations about the tests available. Based on their own experiences, people interviewed offered valuable suggestions on how to get an accurate diagnosis.

Vojdani emphasized that the test results can't simply give you a definite yes or no answer. He explained that a diagnosis should be based on blood serum testing, a person's medical history, and a symptom questionnaire. "Any one of these is not enough," he said. Vojdani also noted that his lab itself does not diagnose Candida overgrowth; it leaves the clinical diagnosis up to each individual doctor.

Broughton said he would recommend the blood serum test to physicians: "The test is inexpensive, reliable, and easy to take." He added that the test also provides a confirmation for a localized infection. When antibodies are interpreted separately without the immune complex, they are not conclusive of Candida overgrowth but can indicate localized yeast infection. "Physicians have comfort levels with antibodies," continued Broughton. "They offer a good history, and a lot of doctors like the antibodies." With these tests, "you get the best of both worlds. The test is very comprehensive and gives the clinician the information he needs to know."

Richard Lord, M.D., the technical director of MetaMetrix Laboratory in Norcross, Georgia, said Candida tests are an issue where there are a lot of opinions. Dr. Lord has worked at MetaMetrix for six years and said when testing for Candida overgrowth, he would first recommend the blood serum test be performed. "It's a really good beginning point to see how the immune system is responding to Candida." He said the serum test is a good reference mark to have at the various stages of a patient's case. Dr. Lord suggested that the physician may want to have stool tests performed after blood tests have been done. When Candida is localized in the gut, it shows up in the stool test. So even though Candida antibodies may not be affecting the system and showing up in the blood, there still may be overgrowth in the gut.

Broughton reports while his lab doesn't track how many of the tests for Candida overgrowth come back positive, an informal study revealed 95 percent of the people who report symptoms to their doctor had increased immune complex tests for Candida. Out of the increased complex group, a full 100 percent responded to treatment. Of the patients with normal immune complexes, only 5 percent respond to treatment, which means the test is sensitive and lacks a false-negative results problem.

Stool Tests

Although there is the possibility of getting a negative stool-test result even when there is an overgrowth of Candida, the tests are a valuable resource. According to research published by Great Smokies regarding which diagnostic tests are the most effective, cultures are a standard means of determining possible overgrowth, colonization, or infection of bacterial or fungal organisms in patients. Cultures also allow for the identification of many organisms at the same time and can help determine whether the infection is equally spread throughout the sample. Great Smokies refers to CRC as yeast-related complex because their diagnostic tests find that Candida isn't the only clinically significant yeast. In order to be as accurate as possible, this chapter will use their term when discussing their research and test results.

One study performed by Great Smokies investigated whether or not people who reported yeast-related complex symptoms actually tested positively for yeast overgrowth. It found that 82 percent of those who had symptoms also had yeast overgrowth in their stool cultures. Among the patients who did not have yeast-related complex symptoms, only 6.4 percent had yeast overgrowth. Given their findings, Great Smokies concluded the fecal yeast culture is highly sensitive and specific, accurately detects yeast overgrowth, and can be used to effectively monitor patients' improvements. Plus, as Dr. James said earlier, stool tests also measure many different health variables and give the physician a wide range of information about the patient's overall health.

Although cultures do sometimes test negatively even though there actually is an overgrowth of Candida, the other two common Candida tests performed by Great Smokies (serum and parasite) can correct that problem. The problem with cultures is that the yeast cells that show up in stool samples are sometimes dead. And since you can't grow live yeast cells from dead ones, a stool culture occasionally produces negative results. Dr James assures patients, however, that if there is yeast overgrowth, both the serum and parasite exams will find it. The parasite exam inspects the stool samples microscopically and looks for and reports on several factors, one of which is dead yeast cells. "If you're really looking for yeast, it's helpful to do all the tests," said Dr. James.

Not only do the sickest patients with confirmed yeast overgrowth sometimes have stool samples that test negatively for yeast overgrowth, many healthy people without Candida-related problems actually do have a limited amount of Candida in their stool. In addition to complicating the diagnostic procedure, this phenomenon is significant for other reasons as well. One concern is that this paradox adds to doubts of those who question the validity of CRC. In her essay "The Paradox of Negative Stool Cultures for Yeasts in Symptomatic Yeast and Mold Allergy Patients," Elizabeth Naugle says, "A major problem in diagnosing gut yeast overgrowth . . . is that the sickest patients usually have *negative* stool cultures for this common organism, whereas healthy controls are often carriers of Candida with *positive* stool cultures. This paradox contributes significantly to the controversy surrounding this 'disputed undiagnosis.'" Naugle is the president of the Candida & Dysbiosis Information Foundation (CDIF) located in College Station, Texas.

The findings of a team of scientists at the University of Ferrara in Italy, which were published in a 1988 article in the medical journal *Digestion*, suggest another reason negative test results are important: the dead Candida cells that cause negative results may be responsible for some of the symptoms associated with CRC. The authors, Caselli et al., had been investigating whether or not large amounts of dead *Candida albicans* cells were responsible for two symptoms associated with irritable bowel syndrome. The researchers concluded that in the absence of other possible causes, the large amounts of dead Candida cells were responsible for chronic recurrent diarrhea and possibly abdominal cramps.

Based on his research that an inhibiting factor found in the rectal mucus of patients is responsible for negative stool cultures, Leo Galland, M.D., has suggested an alternative method to test for the presence of Candida. Dr. Galland reports that even though his sickest patients often have negative stool results, if he takes a rectal swab sample and immediately puts it under a microscope without a fixative (which destroys the cell walls, making the test useless) he can see the yeasts. He advises that because the yeast is buried fairly deeply, it is necessary when taking the rectal swab to scrape the membranes hard enough to cause bleeding to get a correct sample. To support his theory that an inhibiting factor is found in the rectal membrane, Dr. Galland performed an experiment where he took culture plates infused with Candida and then added dots of rectal mucus taken from patients. The Candida organisms failed to grow near the rectal mucus, which shows that some as yet unknown repressing mechanism seems to be at work.

At this point serum tests and Great Smokies's comprehensive digestive stool analysis seem to be the most reliable forms of testing for Candida overgrowth and for helping determine how the patient's body is reacting to Candida. Although no one yet knows for sure why some stool samples may test negatively for Candida, since they provide both doctor and patient with valuable information, they should still be performed when possible.

Choosing Your Doctor

Choose your doctor or health-care provider both deliberately and carefully. It is important to have a doctor who can address both your physical and emotional needs, one who is both a capable medical technician and a good listener. Most people would agree that compassion, understanding, sensitivity, empathy, honesty, and genuine concern about patients and their needs are requisite qualities for good physicians. You probably also want a doctor you can feel comfortable discussing your problems and concerns with.

Finding a physician with these qualities is especially important for the CRC patient. Fungal conditions in general require a longer recovery time than bacterial infections, and CRC is no exception. Because this illness can take months or even years to get under control, CRC patients need to work closely and comfortably with their doctors. These patients must meet with their doctors often to tailor treatment programs to meet their needs at the different stages of recovery. Because this condition can be both confusing and at times overwhelming, the best physician should provide not just information and guidance, but also support and encouragement. Tell your doctor what you require, and if he or she does not seem interested in working with you to meet your needs, find another physician. Don't settle for a doctor who provides less than what you need and deserve.

The impact of a physician on the recovery of his or her patient is tremendous and cannot be denied. As Christiane Northrup, M.D., writes in her book *Women's Bodies, Women's Wisdom*:

> Health care providers must be aware of how powerful their words are. The cloak of the shaman rests on their shoulders whether they realize it or not. Their words have the power to heal or to destroy—partly because of the vulnerability associated with illness and with our bodies. Professionals' words must be truthful and at the same time chosen to support healing.

The authority and power given to doctors in the United States are far more than those given to members of any other profession. Many patients never ask questions or tell their doctors when they aren't meeting their needs. Going to a doctor and putting yourself in the role of patient isn't always easy. When discussing the experience of women as patients, John M. Smith, M.D., writes in his book *Women and Doctors* that a patients role is built around vulnerability and a lack of control. There is "a degree of physical and emotional exposure that is hard to tolerate even in a relationship with a friend or relative, much less with a physician who is neither," he says. For these reasons, it is very important to find a physician who respects you and is sensitive to your vulnerability.

While it is your responsibility to set the tone for the relationship with your health-care provider, it is also up to your doctor to participate equally and make the experience a satisfying one. Your quality of life and your health are at risk. And remember, you are paying your doctor to look after you, not the other way around. Because of our vulnerable role in the doctor/patient relationship, we sometimes forget that we are also paying customers with the right to demand proper service. Too often patients view kindness and genuine concern as unexpected bonuses instead of the basic level of care we deserve. If you aren't satisfied with your present doctor, don't hesitate to consider finding a new one. There are many physicians out there who would be more than happy to work with you in your search to improve your health.

After finding the best doctor possible who can meet your needs, your next goal should be to establish a positive relationship with her. Unfortunately, some difficulties may exist in the quest to build a relationship with your physician, but recognizing these difficulties is the first step in overcoming them. And as the People's Medical Society (the nation's largest consumer health-advocacy organization) writes, "It's not enough to know that problems can arise in the doctor/patient relationship, the real skill is in correcting the minor problem before it turns into a bigger problem."

Changing Doctors: A Difficult but Sometimes Necessary Task

No one will disagree that changing doctors isn't easy, but if the circumstances merit a change, it may be necessary. In *Every Woman's Health*, Frances Drew, M.D., compares changing doctors to a divorce and concludes that patients should get out of bad relationships as soon as possible. "Everyone knows that marriage is easier than divorce and that many marriages are sustained on inertia rather than on compatibility or love," writes Dr. Drew. She also recommends making sure the office of your old physician sends the office of your new physician a copy of your records; no amount of embarrassment should prevent you from getting this information into the hands of your new physician. Your health and satisfaction as a patient are more important than worrying about slighting a physician.

In its health bulletin on how to choose a doctor, the People's Medical Society comments on when patients should switch doctors and lists seven warning signals you should heed, with the first being overcrowded waiting rooms. "You and twenty-two of the doctor's closest friends show up for the first appointment at 8 A.M. Overbooking may be fine for the airlines, but it shouldn't fly in your doctor's office." Two more warning signals are excessive waiting time and being hurried through appointments. The People's Medical Society suggests calling ahead and asking for an approximate waiting time to decrease the amount of time you spend in the waiting room. Two more things to watch out for are unavailability of the doctor and lack of communication. Both interfere with your ability to get necessary medical care. Finally, be wary of fee increases and of being refused access to your medical records. You have every right to have copies of and access to your medical records.

How Changing Attitudes May Affect Your Relationship with Your Doctor

Changing attitudes in society can both help and hinder your attempt to develop a relationship with your doctor. The traditional roles of patient and physician have been changing for more than forty years now. Physicians are no longer the sole guardians of health or medical information: they are now merely players in the game. Since Dr. Benjamin Spock's first book on parenting was published, patients, particularly women, have been given more responsibility in overseeing their health and that of their families. Women have been encouraged to be both savvy consumers and informed participants when it comes to managing their health. Through television, newspapers, and women's magazines, women are bombarded with information about how to take charge of their own health. The information provided by the media both responds to and encourages public interest and awareness.

Unfortunately, while these trends toward independence and medical self-care are beneficial to patients, they clash with the traditional authoritarian setting of the doctor's office. These independent attitudes challenge the authority of the physician and may, in your physician's view, make his job harder. Some physicians may unconsciously find patients who offer a self-diagnosis of their illness threatening. Whether your physician is threatened by you or not, don't be afraid to listen to your own feelings and trust your own judgments. Although physicians are trained to diagnose and treat diseases, you better than anyone else know the circumstances of your own health and life. It may take time to find a doctor who is both understanding and familiar with Candida, but one with these qualities will be more than happy to work with you to solve your Candida-related problems.

The changes in attitude haven't been easy on physicians or patients. Research on what causes disease has added to the trend of patient responsibility and awareness. More and more diseases have been found to be related to lifestyle, which is to some degree under the control of the patient. Patients may find it hard to accept responsibility for making difficult changes in their lives and may feel that their physician should be able to fix all their problems. But physicians can no longer take full responsibility for their patient's health, nor can they prescribe miracle drugs or undo decades of unhealthy habits.

Not all physicians are critical of the increasing independence of patients; in fact, many recognize this change as being beneficial for both patient and physician. As Dr. Drew writes, "Sensing a mounting backlash against the entire profession, doctors are responding (in many cases grudgingly) to the increasing independence of women so that a partnership is established in which both parties profit from the circumstance that the well-informed patient is healthier, recovers faster, and is more gratifying to treat."

Building a Relationship with Your Doctor

A doctor should not resist your attempts to build a relationship. If she does, be on your guard. Unfortunately, because they are busy and see dozens of patients every day, physicians sometimes try to interact with their patients no more than is absolutely necessary. Although doctors have busy schedules, you have the right to expect your physician to treat you as an individual patient and to talk with you about your problem. In many cases, physicians who regularly treat CRC seem to be more inclined to sit down and work out the solutions to your health problems with you. They are familiar with CRC and know it involves more than a simple exam or prescription. In general, doctors who treat CRC tend to be more patient-oriented, which makes sense when you consider they are treating a medical condition criticized by some of their colleagues.

In her exceptional book *How to Talk to Your Doctor: The Questions to Ask,* Janet R. Maurer, M.D., suggests patients approach their physicians with these common sense principles in mind:

- Make it clear to your doctor that you are interested in learning about your illness.

- Take notes and ask your physician if he has any printed versions of the information he is explaining to you.

- Organize your thoughts and questions before seeing your doctor.

- Volunteer any facts or information you think might have been forgotten or overlooked.

- When asking questions make them as specific as possible.

- Come to terms with your anxieties and your fear of the unknown; often the truth is not as bad as you think it will be.

- If you don't understand what your doctor is telling you, ask for a simpler or clearer explanation. If you leave your physician's office without a full understanding of the information your physician has given you, you are doing a disservice both to yourself and your doctor.

- On later visits, don't be shy about asking your physician to repeat vital information and to explain to you her evaluation of your progress.

- Don't ask questions that have no answers. While your physician will help you to the best of her ability, she cannot give you certainties or make future predictions, such as how long you will have to take medications or how long your recovery will take.

The first step in developing a good relationship with your physician is to be prepared with information on your symptoms and medical history when you visit your doctor. It is also important to give your physician feedback on whether or not he is adequately helping you. Remember to present both yourself and your needs to your doctors: assuming they lack supernatural powers, it is impossible for them to know your needs and expectations without you first telling them. If you do decide to change doctors, let your doctor know you are seeking the services he did not provide elsewhere. You deserve a doctor you can work with and respect. As Dr. Smith writes, "There is no more reason to provide income for a bad doctor than to pay for rotten apples at the market. A great deal has been accomplished in our country through aggressive consumerism, and the medical profession can be made responsive to its consumers in the same fashion."

Although communicating your expectations to your doctor may be difficult, it is an important part of building a relationship and your best hope for getting the most out of your medical visits. If your doctor doesn't see you as a real person then he may not invest as much of himself into the relationship as you would like. And it goes without saying that since your physician is half of this partnership, you should try to get to know him as a person and recognize his expectations as well.

Getting to Know a New Doctor

Before you schedule an appointment with a new doctor, you have every right to ask for the following information: the physician's qualifications and specialties; the fees charged by that office; whether or you will have to pay the doctor and wait for reimbursement from the insurance company or whether the doctor applies for reimbursement; and how long the initial appointment takes and how you should prepare for it. You may also want to discuss the physician's office hours, and if you decide to stay with this physician, you should ask how to reach her in case of an emergency.

If at all possible, go for your first visit when you are feeling your best so your physician can have a normal standard to measure any future problems against. On that first visit you should also either bring all your medications (both nonprescription and prescription) with you, or bring a detailed list that includes the recommended dosage of each medication. Also bring a copy of your medical records and be prepared to discuss whatever health problems you are having.

Since you are a first-time patient, the doctor should make the effort to get to know you and make you feel comfortable. The doctor should also get to know you both physically and personally since both aspects of you are important to your health. If the visit requires a physical exam the physician should also meet you and first talk to you before you undress. Dr. Smith notes, "Meeting you for the first time *after* you have undressed shows a lack of sensitivity that probably will be reflected in everything else he does." If the nurse or assistant asks you to undress before you meet the doctor, ask to first meet the doctor with your clothing on. If the assistant or doctor refuses or becomes angry, leave. "Anything that puts you on unequal footing with the doctor is inappropriate. There is no reason for you to undress for a complete stranger, which the doctor will be until you have had a chance to meet and talk," Dr. Smith adds.

At the initial meeting try to accomplish two goals: allow the doctor to get to know you and your expectations and find out the physician's personal style, attitudes, and expectations of you. This would also be a good time to ask questions about your future working relationship; for instance, is the doctor willing to be your primary-care physician? You will also want to know who treats her patients when she is unavailable, whether or not the office will return phone calls, and how you will get to see the doctor if you have an emergency or if you have a critical problem that needs to be treated on extremely short notice. Of course, your doctor's answers are important, but what is more important is her attitude and willingness to discuss these concerns with you.

It is up to each one of us to demand fair and individual treatment. As Dr. Smith reminds us, "Don't give your trust until it is earned, and don't accept insensitive treatment, demeaning procedures, or lack of personal regard. Women have, in some measure, helped create the bad practices that exist by accepting them. The practices are not unchangeable. . . . They [women] must cease to reward bad behavior."

What You Should Expect from Your Doctor
First and foremost, you have the right to expect help and guidance from your doctor. Why else would you be there if not to ask for help getting through an illness and guidance on how to recover both emotionally and physically?

There are also several more specific things you should feel within your rights to expect from your doctor. In her book *How to Talk to Your Doctor*, Dr. Maurer lists your rights as a patient:

- To be seen by the doctor within a reasonable amount of time. Dr. Maurer suggests thirty minutes as a not unreasonable amount of time to wait.

- To be given as much information as you wish about your medical condition.

- To be given enough time to ask questions about your concerns.

- To be given simple and straightforward answers to your questions. If your doctor is extremely busy at that moment, ask whether he would like you to schedule another appointment in the very near future.

- To be allowed reasonable access to your physician, which is something you and your physician should agree on as soon as possible.

- To be able to participate in the decisions regarding your medical care.

- To be able to decide who other than your physician will have access to your medical records and information about your health.

Patients also have certain responsibilities to help safeguard their health. These obligations include the following:

- Asking questions.

- Asking your doctor for a clearer explanation when you do not understand what he tells you.

- Knowing the office hours of your physician and his policy for contacting him after hours.

- Changing physicians if there is an unresolvable problem.

- Following the prescribed therapy your physician recommends. If you are having doubts about the treatment or cannot complete it because of side effects from the medication (or for any other reason), do not hesitate to let your physician know your problems or concerns.

The act of going to the doctor has changed. Doctors are no longer commanding and authoritarian. They no longer possess knowledge available to only a select few. Medicine has become more of a helping profession in response to the expectations of patients. Although the advice presented above may not apply to every relationship with every physician, it should give you an idea of your rights and what you can reasonably expect from your doctor.

What Your Doctor Should Expect from You
Just as you should expect certain behaviors from your physician, she has the right to expect some from you. Although many of these

requests should fall into the category of common courtesy, they still deserve discussion. Physicians have the right to expect the following from you:

- To be notified as soon as possible if you will be unable to make your appointment.
- To be notified if you are going to be late for your appointment.
- To have the fee for the visit paid before you leave the office, unless prior arrangements have been made.

Some behaviors not only show respect and consideration for your doctor, but also affect your health. Doctors should expect the following:

- To be told all the information relevant to your present illnesses and overall health.
- To be told the truth about your compliance with the prescribed treatment, whether the treatment is formal such as medication, or informal such as increased exercise and better nutrition.
- To be given enough time to perform tests and evaluations before making a concrete diagnosis.
- To be notified of the side effects of medications, or any changes in your health.
- To be told if you have sought a second opinion and are currently following the recommendations of another physician.
- To not act in a manner he or she thinks may not be in your best interests.
- To not be expected to be able to predict side effects of a medication; medications have different side effects on each patient.
- To not be expected to predict the outcome of a medical condition or to predict exactly how long recovery will take.

The best possible relationship between a physician and patient is one of mutual effort, which then provides mutual gain. While very few patients would deliberately act rudely toward their physician, they may not perceive withholding information or taking part in any of the other actions listed above as harmful or discourteous, when in fact doing so may affect both their relationship with their physician and their health.

Finding a Physician Who Treats Candida

Unfortunately, finding a doctor who is knowledgeable about Candida and treats CRC is not an easy task. Although some organizations and books, including this one, do publish lists of doctors, this is no guarantee the doctors listed will meet your needs, or even, in some cases, treat Candida. One organization that publishes a list of nutritionally oriented health-care givers is the Price-Pottenger Nutrition Foundation, a nonprofit educational corporation. For a list of health-care givers in your area, send a self-addressed stamped envelope and a $6 donation to the Price-Pottenger Nutrition Foundation, P.O. Box 2614, La Mesa, CA 91943-2614. Please specify the state for which you need a listing and, if your city is on the border of another state, the name of your neighboring state.

Finding the right physician to help with your Candida may not be easy. One suggestion is to ask the staff of your local health food store if they know doctors who treat Candida in the area. Another is to try to reach other CRC patients in your community who can share their experiences and advice about local doctors. One possible way of finding other CRC patients is to see if your local health food store has a bulletin board or place for posting messages and to place a sign about CRC or even about Chronic Fatigue Syndrome. You can also check with local doctors who practice alternative medicine, such as chiropractors, nutritionists, or homeopathic or naturopathic physicians to see if they know who in the area may be treating CRC.

If you are unable to find a doctor who is familiar with Candida and your present doctor is open-minded enough to listen to you and help you try to treat your CRC, you will have to decide whether or not you want to receive treatment from her. Although any doctor can prescribe medications and educate herself on a medical condition, her unfamiliarity with CRC means she isn't well versed in the specifics of treatment, such as proper dosages or administration of anti-Candida medications. If you are having problems finding a physician familiar with CRC, you might be wise to stay under the care of your present doctor so that you have some medical guidance, but consider continuing your search until you are able to find someone more experienced to help you recover from CRC.

You and Your Pharmacist

Medications play a large role in our lives. In fact, Americans spend $40 billion a year on prescription and nonprescription medications. Consequently, our relationships with our pharmacists take on great significance. A pharmacist's many roles include medication expert, medication advisor, and medication counselor. In the last twenty-five years, the local pharmacy has expanded its role in the health-care delivery system from simply preparing and dispensing medications to providing a wide range of patient-oriented services that help patients get the maximum possible benefits from their medications.

While there are several reasons to choose your pharmacist carefully, two of the best are emphasized in a health bulletin on how to choose your pharmacist issued by the People's Medical Society:

> More than just a pill counter, the community pharmacist is the most readily accessible health-care professional most of us have—no appointment is needed. The pharmacist is a highly trained drug expert who probably knows more than your own physician about the relative benefits and risks of various drugs. And with today's medications more complex and, in some cases, more potent, and with drug prescribing on the increase, you need to find a competent and communicative pharmacist—now more than ever.

Many people tend to have better relationships with their pharmacists than with their physicians. There are several possible reasons for this. One reason might be that the setting is less authoritarian. In addition, pharmacists know less about the deep dark secrets patients feel obligated to tell their doctors. And since patients don't directly pay pharmacists for their advice, patients' expectations are lower, so there may be less tension between customer and pharmacist. As compared to doctors, pharmacists are also perceived by patients as being more caring and easier to talk to.

Taking full advantage of your relationship with your pharmacist and asking questions are extremely important. According to the People's Medical Society, "Communicating about medications must become a routine part of any encounter where medications are prescribed or dispensed. In short, you are shopping for a pharmacist who is comfortable with and adept at his/her role of patient educator." As we all know, clear and confident communication is the key to any good relationship. This is especially true in your relationship with your pharmacist.

Medication counseling (by pharmacists or physicians) has also been found to help patients better stick to their medication regimens, according to a 1994 article in the *American Journal of Hospital Pharmacy*. More than two thousand patients were asked whether or not they received medication counseling and the effects it had on them. Patients who received some counseling, either by their physician or pharmacist, were more likely to have taken their medication. The survey results were not surprising but are certainly worth noting:

Counseled by:	Took medication exactly as prescribed:
Pharmacist	96 percent
Physician	89 percent
Both pharmacist and physician	93 percent
Neither pharmacist nor physician	77 percent

Pharmacists are there not only to answer questions about prescription medications, but also to help with nonprescription medicines, which, even though they are available without a prescription, are still very powerful and even potentially dangerous. Choose your pharmacist as carefully as you would your doctor. Don't choose a pharmacist based on location, but rather based on how attentive he is to your needs and the kind of relationship you have developed or believe you can develop. Don't hesitate to ask your pharmacist any questions; your pharmacist's role as medication counselor is one of his most important functions.

Many consumers feel more comfortable speaking with their pharmacist than their doctors. A survey conducted in 1993 by the National Prescription Buyers produced the following conclusions:

- During a six-month period, 85 percent of people surveyed said they speak with their pharmacist regarding their medications.

- When it comes to initiating conversations, the numbers are almost equally split with patients taking the initiative 45 percent of the time and pharmacists taking it 48 percent of the time. According to the statistics available, pharmacists are starting conversations more frequently than five years ago.

- Patients are more likely to discuss prescription medications with their pharmacists than any other topic. A reported 67 percent of patients asked pharmacists about prescription medicines, 64 percent asked about nonprescription medicines, and 47 percent asked for advice on how to treat an illness or injury.

- Pharmacists are viewed by the majority of patients as the primary source of information on medications. A full 56 percent of those surveyed reported that their primary advisors on medications were their pharmacists rather than their doctors. Five years ago only 44 percent of patients chose their pharmacists over their doctors for this information.

Just as in your relationship with your physician, it is important to realize that while the pharmacist can provide the services and help that you need, it is up to you to take advantage of these services if and when you need them. If you don't ask questions, the pharmacist will assume you are familiar with your medication and do not need his help. When discussing your medical problems with your pharmacist, it is your responsibility to provide the following information:

- What drugs you are currently taking, both prescription and nonprescription.
- Any problem you might be having with your medications.
- Which, if any, medications you are allergic to.
- If you are or think you may be pregnant.
- The most up-to-date information on your medical condition.

The People's Medical Society says that a good pharmacist does more than read prescriptions and fill little brown bottles. A good pharmacist is "willing and eager to expand the pharmacist's role, beyond that of a 'pill counter,' to a recognized member of the health-care team and a drug information specialist." A good pharmacist also keeps family information records; advises on *exactly* how to take your medications, both prescription and nonprescription; answers your questions; and advises you when you should seek the help of a doctor.

The American Pharmaceutical Association recommends all patients ask their pharmacists these ten questions:

- What is the name of the medication and what is it supposed to do?
- When and how do I take it?
- How long should I take it?
- Does this medication contain anything that could cause an allergic reaction?
- Should I avoid alcohol, any other medications, foods, or activities?
- Should I expect any side effects? What should I do if I experience side effects?
- Is there a generic version of the medication my doctor has prescribed?
- What if I forget to take my medication?
- Is it safe to become pregnant or to breast-feed while taking this medication?

- How should I store my medications?

Other questions you should ask are:

- Can I get a refill? If so, when should I get one?
- Is there any written information about this medicine?
- Are there any long-term, harmful side effects of this medicine?
- What should I do if someone else takes my medication or if I accidentally take too many pills or too much medicine?

There are also a few guidelines you should follow to ensure that you get the most help from your pharmacist and take your medications with the greatest level of safety:

- Know the correct medical name for your illness or condition.
- Go to one pharmacy so all your records will be in one place.
- Read the directions. If there is any reason you cannot read them, have someone read the directions to you.
- Ask the pharmacist to explain the medicine's directions if you do not understand them.
- Take notes on what you are told about your medications.
- Make sure your medications are clearly labeled and identified.
- Call your pharmacist if you have any questions no matter how small or silly they seem to you. Your health is your most important asset.
- Finish all the medication prescribed by your doctor. Don't assume that because the symptoms stop or that you feel better you should discontinue your medication.

There are also some things you should never do:

- Do not put one medication into a bottle labeled for another medication.
- Do not keep medications and self-prescribe them if you believe you have the same illness or condition again. Only your doctor and pharmacist should make that decision.
- Do not share medications with your friends or family. Each patient is different and may need a different dosage, the medication may be unsuitable for the person, or the person may not even have the illness he thinks he has.

According to the American Pharmaceutical Association, the National Council on Patient Information and Education (NCPIE) estimates that "90 percent of *all drugs* [that includes prescription and nonprescription] are not taken as directed, which costs our nation some 125,000 lives per year and also adds $20 billion to the annual U.S. health care bill."

NCPIE also estimates that 50 percent of all prescription drugs are taken incorrectly. The NCPIE lists five contributing factors to patient noncompliance with directions for prescription medications: poor communication between the patient and the health-care provider; use of multiple health-care providers; inability to take the medication as prescribed; deliberate noncompliance; and altered drug action and response due to advancing age. The repercussions of not taking medications correctly include prolonged illness, avoidable side effects, drug interactions, increased hospitalizations, absences from work, overuse of health-care services, and possibly even death.

Many patients are unaware of what constitutes a moderate or severe side effect. Moderate side effects include mild forms of these problems: nausea, headache, stomach upset, constipation, diarrhea, and dry mouth. Contact your doctor or pharmacist if you have these more serious side effects: fever, skin rash, blood in your urine or stool, any changes in your eyesight or hearing, dizziness, or unusual or sudden pain.

Make sure you understand how your insurance plan covers the costs of your medications. If you have questions, call your pharmacist or your insurance company. If you cannot afford health insurance ask your pharmacist or physician how state agencies may help pay for your prescription medicines.

Although the articles in pharmaceutical journals and pamphlets published by pharmaceutical associations reported positively on the ability to develop a relationship with a pharmacist, do their expectations fit the reality of patient/pharmacist relations? Although most people would like to get to know their pharmacist, both patients and pharmacist are usually too busy to talk to each other unless absolutely necessary. In addition, most pharmacists don't know that much about CRC and may be able to answer only specific questions on the medications used to treat it, but not questions on CRC in general.

Jack Parker, a pharmacist who owns a pharmacy/health food store in upstate New York, said, "I don't think the average pharmacist knows enough about this [CRC]. This is still not a recognized problem." He said he didn't think most pharmacists would have much information or advice to offer CRC patients. "Patients have to help themselves; no one is going to come and prepare meals with them." Nonetheless, it wouldn't hurt to ask your pharmacist if she is familiar with CRC, and you should definitely ask her about any medications you may take to treat it.

How to Read a Prescription

Although your physician fills out your prescriptions for you to pass on to your pharmacist to fill, having some basic knowledge of your physician's intent can help you double-check not only your busy physician, but also your pharmacist. Your medical health is too important to fully leave in the care of others who, although they have your best interests at heart, are busy and may have to field constant interruptions while trying to do a dozen tasks at once.

Too often physicians don't take the time to fully explain what medications they are giving you and why unless you show an interest. Since you may not think of a question until after you've left your doctor's office, the handy chart below may prove to be helpful. Assuming you can decipher your physician's handwriting, the following list gives you an idea of what your physician has written.

WHEN TO TAKE THE MEDICATION:		QUANTITY PRESCRIBED BY DOCTOR:	
ac	before meals	aa	equal amounts of each
ad lib	whenever you want	cc	cubic centimeter
bid	twice a day	dr	dram
pc	after meals	extr	extract
p.r.n.	as needed	gm	gram
qd	every day	gr	grains
qh	every hour	gt	drop
qid	four times a day	mg	milligrams
qs	as much as is sufficient	min	minim, a drop

OTHERS:	
od	right eye
os	left eye
Sig	directions for taking

For many patients getting well often means relying or depending on the advice and knowledge of their physicians and pharmacists. Don't settle for someone who gives less than you need. And once you find your ideal physician or pharmacist, be sure to communicate your need for an equally beneficial relationship.

—7—

The Immune Response

The terrain is everything, the bacteria is nothing.
—Louis Pasteur, quoted by E.D. Hume in *Pasteur Exposed: The False Foundations of Modern Medicine*

Every day inside our bodies, wars are fought, battles won and lost, and prisoners executed. These wars are our immune system in action, destroying invaders and keeping our bodies free of infection. Candida overgrowth and the resulting problems that go along with it occur when our defenses are weak and unable to keep the Candida organism at bay.

Since Candida is not a part of the body, understanding how the body reacts to it is important. "*Candida albicans* is a fungus and, although much evidence indicates that it probably lives within everyone, it nevertheless is a substance foreign to and not a part of the body," writes Dr. Truss. An important detail to remember is that the relationship between Candida and the body's immune system has two important aspects. The first is the way in which the immune system controls (or fails to control) Candida growth. The second is how Candida, if it overcomes the body's defenses, works to further weaken the immune system.

When Immune Defenses Fail

As discussed in previous chapters, use of antibiotics may greatly affect the natural defense mechanisms of the immune system that fight Candida. Antibiotics are believed to inhibit one of our immunological defense mechanisms called "complement." Complement is a group of nine different components (proteins) that are numbered C1 through C9, which attack invading microorganisms. Found in the plasma in our blood, the components of complement react in a definitive sequence, with each component activating each other.

Once activated, complement promotes two processes designed to help the body heal itself: inflammation and phagocytosis. Inflammation is the body's way of isolating and destroying foreign substances such as bacteria. Phagocytosis is simply the destruction of dead cells, foreign substances, or microorganisms. The activation of complement by detection of Candida is an important defense mechanism against Candida. Scientists speculate that antibiotic therapy may inhibit activation of one of the components of complement, C3. Therapeutic concentrations of three frequently prescribed antibiotics, sulfadiazine, tetracycline, and gentamicin, have been shown to inhibit C3. "Failure to activate C3 . . . could in turn lead to decreased resistance to *C. albicans* infection. Such observations could at least partly explain the association between broad spectrum antibiotic therapy and susceptibility to Candida infection," write British scientists J.M.A. Wilton and T. Lehner.

Dr. Truss also notes, "When the immune response is inadequate to meet the challenge of an invading germ, the agent escapes destruction and is able to multiply and persist in the tissues." Once the body's defenses have been overcome by the infection, the immune system stops fighting altogether. Instead of continuing to battle, the T cells (which recognize friendly or unfriendly substances) and B cells (which seek and destroy unfriendly invaders) become unresponsive and permit the infection to persist.

Other factors may also contribute to deficient immune resistance to Candida. As Dr. Truss points out, the ease with which many individuals acquire yeast infections suggests such a genetic weakness in their immune response to this organism. An article published in the *Annals of Internal Medicine* in 1971 discusses the genetic factor in relation to chronic mucocutaneous candidiasis. This disease is an uncommon superficial infection of skin, nails, and mucous membranes throughout the body that usually affects people who already have serious defects in cellular immune function. The authors conclude, "Genetic determinants may have an important role in the development of at least some cases of chronic candidiasis." Although most cases are not genetically linked, the ones that are appear to also be linked to either an acute skin disease called furunculosis or endocrine and ectodermal disease. The term *endocrine* refers to the ductless glands in the body such as thyroid, adrenal, ovaries, and testes. Ectodermal disease concerns three parts of the body: the epidermis (the top layer of skin), the nervous system, and sensory organs.

Further Effects of Candida on the Immune System

So how does Candida affect our immune systems and how does that affect us? Since Candida is suspected as a contributor in so many diseases, a great deal of research has been done on the possible links between Candida and the immune system. In his essay "Chronic Candidiasis and Allergy," George F. Kroker, M.D., discusses three of the current research concepts on Candida and its interference with normal immune mechanisms. The concepts are that Candida alters the T suppressor cells, secretes substances that impair immune function, and interferes with correct Candida-antigen delivery by macrophages (which engulf bad microorganisms) to normal T cells. Dr. Kroker reminds the reader of the overall consequences of Candida-induced depressed cellular immunity. This general weakening of defenses can allow even further Candida colonization and the symptoms that follow.

In a recent medical journal, Steven S. Witkin, Ph.D., from the Cornell University Medical College department of obstetrics and gynecology, discusses defective immune system responses in patients who suffer recurrent candidiasis. Based on his findings, he also concludes that Candida can cause defects in cellular immunity and suggests boosting the immune system's defenses while continuing antifungal therapy.

Since Candida overgrowth is a result of weakened immune functions, treatment should be focused on strengthening the immune system. According to Dr. Truss, "All aspects of treatment have the common goal of allowing the immune system to recover its lost capacity to eradicate the yeast from the tissues, for only this can effectively remove the source of the products so toxic to the tissues and to the immune system itself. The goal of treatment, therefore, is the restoration to its genetically determined maximum of immunologic competence to Candida albicans." Once what has been suppressing the immune system has been determined and addressed and other factors that can cause Candida growth are avoided, the immune system can start to flush itself of the Candida toxins that cause all of the troublesome symptoms.

SUCCESSFUL TREATMENT
OF CRC

—8—

Recovery: The Basics

It is the body which is the hero, not science, not antibiotics, not machines or new devices.
—Ronald J. Glasser, M.D., in *The Body Is the Hero*

The chapters in this book, and in this section in particular, are designed to help patients get their CRC under control both physically and psychologically.

Treating CRC involves more than treating other medical conditions because it requires changing the way you live. Unlike some medical conditions, there is no "cure" or quick fix for CRC. Unless you follow all three important steps—the diet, the antifungal medications, and the additional treatments—recovery will either crawl along at a snail's pace or not occur at all. Of the treatments, the hardest and most important is the Candida control diet. Many patients try to get by without following the diet or by partially following it. By doing so, they prolong their suffering and make recovery an almost impossible goal.

Making the decision to start treating CRC is a big step for some patients. Many patients delay treatment for years or never begin it at all because their hectic lifestyles make it difficult to develop healthy habits. Another reason patients postpone treatment is because we as a society are too used to quick solutions. Once the difficult changes have been made and recovery is underway, a complete return to a former lifestyle that may have included a high-sugar and high-carbohydrate diet, high-stress situations, antibiotics, and birth control pills is impossible. Given this, it is important to fully understand not only what lifestyle adjustments have to be made, but also the reasons behind the necessary changes. The more you understand about how your habits affect your health, the easier it will be for you to stick with your treatment program.

Separate chapters explain the Candida control diet, the medications commonly prescribed for CRC, and the additional and equally important treatments CRC patients use in their struggle toward good health. Another chapter offers advice on what to do if you are not recovering despite having followed the treatments.

Although a full restoration of health will take time (depending on each individual case), the steps toward recovery are straightforward and simple. In fact, the treatment of CRC is similar to its prevention; both involve the avoidance of factors that increase Candida growth and weaken the immune system. All treatments for CRC have two goals: to reduce the amount of Candida in body tissues and to strengthen your weakened immune system until it is once again able to control abnormal growth of Candida. As mentioned previously, the toxins released by Candida into the bloodstream and carried throughout the body are responsible for the symptoms of CRC. Decreasing the amount Candida in the tissues and clearing the Candida products out of the bloodstream reduce or eliminate symptoms. Decreasing the amount of toxins in the body also helps restore proper function of the immune system. Dr. Truss explains in *The Missing Diagnosis*:

> It is the chronic exposure of the white blood cells (and remainder of the immune system) to these yeast products that is thought to induce the loss of immune responsiveness to the fungus. By reducing their exposure to yeast products while at the same time stimulating them with vaccine, we enable the white blood cells to regain their lost ability to react to this fungus and ultimately to eradicate it from the tissues.

One way of reducing the amount of toxins in the body is to avoid the factors known to cause Candida (listed previously in chapter 5). It is especially important to avoid the following:

- A diet high in sugar.
- Antibiotics and birth control pills. Antibiotics should be used only when medically necessary and when you and your doctor have thoroughly discussed all possible alternatives.
- Immunosuppressive drugs, such as cortisone or steroids. Immunosuppressive drugs are used to prevent or suppress inflammation, which is the immune system's reaction to germs or other foreign agents.

- Environmental molds, especially those that CRC patients are frequently sensitive to and that often produce allergic reactions.

Besides avoiding common factors known to cause CRC, patients should adhere to the following basic steps of recovery:

- Stick to the Candida control diet and rotate your foods regularly
- Take antifungal medications. Although some patients wish to avoid medications and try to control CRC strictly through diet, people who do so relapse more often than people who both follow the diet and take antifungal medications.
- Take *Lactobacillus acidophilus* supplements, which will help restore the balance of microorganisms in the body.
- Take nutritional supplements to strengthen the immune system.
- Exercise regularly.
- Reduce stress levels.

It is extremely important to carefully follow the Candida control diet. The diet is by far the most important step of recovery; many patients who have trouble recovering find that it is because they cannot stick to the diet. Staying on the diet may be difficult, but recovery is virtually impossible without strict adherence to it.

One possible treatment used by doctors who treat CRC is the use of yeast vaccines. Yeast vaccines may be used to help stimulate the immune system in the same way vaccinations help children develop immunity to childhood diseases.

Most physicians who treat Candida refer to the diet and medications as a therapeutic trial. If the patient does not show recovery after three to four months, the trial is considered a failure. However, most patients begin to feel better after only several days or weeks. Dr. Remington cautions that some patience is needed. "Remember, too, that candidiasis is a chronic infection, and chronic infections are sometimes slow and difficult to treat. Improvement is often gradual. While you may notice an immediate and dramatic improvement in some of your symptoms, it may take much longer to notice the improvement in others."

Sidney M. Baker, M.D., former director of the Gesell Institute of Human Development in New Haven, Connecticut, has this to say about recovering from CRC, "Eliminating yeasts totally from one's body is neither feasible nor desirable considering that yeasts probably benefit the body when a proper balance exists. Treatment of the yeast problem seeks not the eradication of yeast from the diet or the person, but rather a new relationship between the person and the yeast."

Die-Off: A Common Reaction to Antifungal Treatment

The combination of medication and diet discourages Candida growth and can produce a strong reaction in the patient called "die-off" or the Herxheimer reaction. When die-off occurs, large numbers of Candida organisms die at one time, releasing toxins throughout the body. These toxins are the same ones responsible for the symptoms that characterize CRC. A patient experiencing die-off may exhibit unpleasant symptoms, such as aches, pains, and a general worsening and intensifying of all symptoms.

Physicians don't usually consider die-off symptoms as side effects of the prescribed medication, but rather a positive sign that the treatment plan is working. Die-off symptoms are sometimes interpreted by the patient as a negative reaction to the medication, but they are just an uncomfortable stage of recovery that must be endured before total health can be reached. Die-off symptoms discontinue after several days.

Although there are many factors involved, die-off symptoms are less or more likely to occur depending on the medication your physician prescribes. In general, the azole drugs (Nizerol, Diflucan, and Sporanox) discussed later in this book are less likely to produce as many die-off symptoms as nystatin seems to produce.

Discomfort from a too-rapid die-off can be lessened by following these three steps:

1. Follow the Candida control diet for one or two weeks before taking antifungal medications. When you do start medications, begin at a low dosage and gradually work up to the full dosage. This method keeps die-off at a moderate rate, allowing the body to adjust slowly to the changes occurring because of the antifungal drugs.

2. Take over-the-counter health food store aids. Three readily available remedies that can relieve the discomfort of a too-rapid die-off are buffered vitamin C, activated charcoal, and Alka-Seltzer Gold. Vitamin C helps boost the immune system, and activated charcoal helps by absorbing toxins and lessening die-off reactions. Alka-Seltzer Gold is the same as bi-salts, which are sodium bicarbonate and potassium bicarbonate. Alka-Seltzer Gold is often used for relief of acute food intolerance problems, but should not be overused as it leads to blood-pressure problems in some patients.

In *The Candida Directory and Cookbook*, Helen Gustafson and Maureen O'Shea suggest patients drink grapefruit tea to help relieve die-off symptoms. Because the tea is acidic, it helps relieve die-off symptoms by neutralizing the alkaline Candida by-products. Grapefruit tea can be made by boiling a section of an organic grapefruit (leave the skin on) in a nonmetallic pot with two pints of purified water for ten minutes. With the pot lid on, let the tea cool to room temperature, then strain it through a sieve. Gustafson and O'Shea recommend several glasses of grapefruit tea every day.

3. Use common sense methods to boost your immune system and do not participate in activities that will further tax your body. Some techniques include getting enough rest, avoiding stress as much as possible, avoiding foods and substances you know you are allergic to, and eating well-balanced, nourishing meals.

It is important to be patient with yourself and your body as you begin the slow trip back to good health. Fungal infections are different from most other infections, and they can take more time and more patience than other illnesses you may have encountered. It isn't a question of whether or not your health will improve, but more a question of when and how.

—9—

The Candida Control Diet

The sick man is not to be pitied who has a cure
up his sleeve.
—Michel de Montaigne in *Essays*

He that takes medicine and neglects to diet
himself wastes the skill of the physician.
—Chinese proverb

For some people, sticking to the Candida control diet is the most difficult part of treating CRC. Many patients are willing to try everything but the diet. As a society, we are accustomed to solving our health problems with pills and quick fixes, not by changing our diets and the way we live.

As we know, CRC is a chronic illness, but there is a proven treatment, and most are able to recover from CRC or at least keep it under control. Even though the diet is strict (and probably requires big changes from you), try not to view it as a restriction, but rather as your best possibility for recovery. Try to view the diet with what Dr. Sehnert calls the Rev. Schuller philosophy: "You are not giving up *anything*—you are gaining *everything*."

Although the Candida control diet could be divided into simple rules and procedures, when you consider the impact food has on our lives, there is really nothing simple about the Candida control diet. The diet is more than lists of acceptable or unacceptable foods; it affects the food choices of family members, changes the way you shop at the grocery store, and influences your choices when you socialize or eat in restaurants.

101

As you follow the diet, keep these three overall suggestions in mind:

- *Tailor your diet* to fit how your CRC is affecting you, particularly during stage two and after. This doesn't mean you can eat whatever you want at any given time; it means in order to recover you need to listen to and work with your body.
- *Rotate your foods* so you eat a variety of foods. Have each item every four to seven days. This is important for two reasons: it will help you identify your allergies and will keep you from becoming addicted to certain foods.
- *Be sure to eat enough food.* One of the purposes of the diet is to heal the body through nutrition, and this requires getting enough nutrients to help your body help itself. Dr. Remington stresses the importance of getting adequate nutrition: "We've seen many people who have developed candidiasis either during or after a restrictive, low-calorie diet." Not getting enough food can cause many of the same symptoms associated with CRC.

Although you have fewer food choices than before you started the diet, there are a great many interesting foods you can still eat. In *The Candida Directory and Cookbook*, Helen Gustafson and Maureen O'Shea make the point that a diet designed to control Candida doesn't have to be bland, just careful. Dr. Lorenzani writes, "Your starvation is not an issue. Starvation of Candida is the issue."

The Two Stages of the Candida Control Diet

The Candida control diet is divided into two stages. In order to deprive the Candida in your body of what it needs to survive, stage one, which has to be strictly followed, eliminates a large variety of foods.

Stage one forbids three types of foods: all foods that will produce allergic reactions, foods that encourage Candida growth, and foods with empty calories and no nutritional value. During stage one, try limiting your carbohydrate intake to between seventy and one hundred grams a day. To be on the safe side, restrict your carbohydrate intake as best you can for the first two to three weeks.

Stage one can last anywhere from four weeks to several months. Its exact duration depends on how your body responds and how quickly you begin to heal. Pay attention to your body. When you feel that your health has improved enough to add foods to your diet, do so. But be careful. If your body signals you that it's not ready with a worsening of symptoms, wait a bit longer.

Stage two prescribes the gradual addition of certain foods to your diet, though many products should still be avoided. This stage of the Candida control diet ends when you feel you have fully regained your health. However, you will most likely always need to be careful what you eat so that you can maintain your new health. There are certain foods that you should probably avoid even after you complete the diet, and they are listed separately from the foods recommended for stage one and stage two later in this chapter. The number of items from this list you will have to permanently avoid eating and the frequency that you eat certain other foods all depend on your individual health. Some people may feel strong enough to tolerate an occasional splurge on cookies. Others may become ill after drinking one soft drink. The important thing is to listen to your body when making these health decisions.

Find and Eliminate Foods You Are Allergic To

Food allergies and sensitivities are part of the many symptoms that characterize CRC. One reason CRC patients develop allergies and sensitivities is because of the "leaky gut" problem explained in chapter 3. Candida overgrowth in the gut (intestine) weakens the mucus membrane, which allows undigested food particles to travel into the bloodstream. The immune system believes these food particles are dangerous microorganisms and attacks them.

Food allergies can be divided into two categories: immediate, or type 1 allergies, in which the reaction comes shortly after the food has been eaten, and delayed, or type 2 allergies, in which the reaction is later and harder to pinpoint. Dairy products, wheat, corn, soy, citrus fruits, yeast, eggs, chocolate, and peanuts are likely candidates for allergies. CRC patients are also commonly allergic to artificial colors and preservatives.

Additional Advice on Staying Healthy

As mentioned above, even after your health is on steady ground, you will need to eat a healthy diet that strictly limits certain foods. You can *occasionally* indulge yourself, but when you eat certain foods, you will notice a return of your previous symptoms.

As the name indicates, the Candida control diet keeps the Candida in your body under control. Whether or not you will regain your health is up to you and how seriously you take your health problems. You must strictly adhere to the diet for as long as you have symptoms and carefully watch what you eat for the rest of your life.

In *Who Killed Candida?*, Vicki Glassburn, a former CRC patient, lists three golden rules staying well after having recovered from Candida. She recommends that if your original symptoms return, go back to strictly following the diet. She also reminds patients that being healthy depends on sticking closely to the food restrictions associated with the diet designed to control Candida. And finally, she adds this important advice: "The immune system takes many, many months to truly rebuild, even though one feels well before then. It is important to give the body time to recover, then always treat it with healthy respect, kindness, and regularity."

Many patients report that after having followed the Candida control diet and having recovered from CRC, their health is the best it has ever been in their lives. Hopefully this will be true for you as well and will encourage you to continue to improve your health through nutrition. In *Candida Albicans*, Leon Chaitow, D.O., N.D., writes that for some patients the new sense of well-being that comes with recovery motivates them to maintain healthy diet and lifestyle habits. In addition, some even develop a taste for the foods on the Candida control diet and stick to it as much for pleasure as for health.

After all, Dr. Chaitow writes, the Candida control diet is not a life sentence. Although you will need to avoid eating foods with refined white sugar, a great many other sweeteners and other tasty foods are available.

It is extremely important to avoid sugar as much as possible, and this includes a variety of medications, vitamins, and oral care products that contain sugar. Read labels carefully and choose only sugar-free products.

The Diet

This section contains specific information on what CRC patients should and should not eat while following the Candida control diet. Remember, the diet is divided into two stages to allow the body to become accustomed to the changes taking place and to help you determine which foods you can or cannot tolerate. The Candida control diet has two purposes: to avoid foods that increase Candida growth and to avoid foods that cause allergic reactions (such as those that contain mold or yeast). Although these are the main goals of the diet, other goals are to encourage healthy eating and to heal a body overtaxed by Candida through nutrition.

In essence, the Candida control diet is a low-fat, sugar-free, high-complex carbohydrate diet. Besides discouraging Candida growth, this type of diet encourages good health.

Foods to Eat during Stage One of the Diet (or Any Time)

The foods you eat must be nutritious, wholesome, and fresh (organic if possible) because these qualities ensure that your body will receive the most nutrients possible. The ultimate goal of any and all treatments for CRC is to help the body help itself. As your health is restored, your immune system will become stronger and will be able to work against the Candida overgrowth. The best foods to help you regain your health contain complex carbohydrates and unrefined carbohydrates and include vegetables and whole grains. The foods must be as pure and unprocessed as possible. Be sure to read all labels carefully before buying anything.

Foods and categories of foods that you are encouraged to eat during any stage of the diet include the following:

Agar-Agar, another name for seaweed, is a tasty and healthy treat.

Baked goods are allowed if they have been leavened with baking powder or baking soda. Corn tortillas are safe because they rarely contain yeast, but be sure to read the label. One way to both avoid yeast and increase your vitamin and mineral intake is to avoid regular flour and use stone-ground cornmeal, whole grain products, or whole wheat flour.

Baked goods with yeast are permitted if you can tolerate them. In *The Yeast Connection*, Dr. Crook interviews John. W. Rippon, Ph.D., an authority on yeasts and molds. Dr. Rippon says that just because patients have problems with Candida, they may not necessarily be allergic to all yeast, and not all yeasts are bad. Drs. Rippon and Crook recommend that patients avoid yeasty foods in the very beginning of their treatment, or at least until they can determine whether or not yeasty foods will provoke allergies. If you can tolerate yeasts other than Candida, you may want to frequently rotate them along with other potentially problematic foods.

Beverages, such as filtered or purified water, are highly recommended. To liven up your water, try adding a touch of lime or lemon juice. Other beverages that are allowed are unsweetened cranberry juice made from concentrate, Perrier, seltzer water, soda water, soy or almond milk, and vegetable juices (except carrot or beet), but only if they are fresh and without additives. You may be able to tolerate a coffee substitute that does not contain sugar, malt (which is a sugar), or additives.

Brown rice is a healthy and safe food, but be sure to buy real brown rice and not an instant or flavored version.

Butter, unsalted, is allowed but only in moderation. Healthier alternatives are clarified butter (see recipe under "Cooking Tips" section), and nut spreads such as almond or cashew butter.

Crackers that are yeast- and sugar-free, and preferably made of whole wheat, are healthy snacks.

Grapefruit is allowed, if you can tolerate it.

Legumes, such as beans (including adzuki, anasazi, black, cannellini, fava, great northern, kidney, lentil, lima, mung, navy, northern, pinto, red, soy, and string), lentils, and peas, such as black-eyed peas and chickpeas are allowed.

Lemon and lime juices are permitted and can be used to liven up water or mixed with oil as a salad dressing.

You may or may not be able to tolerate **melons** such as cantaloupe, honeydew, and watermelon. Because of their porous skins, melons are candidates for mold, but if you carefully wash the melons before cutting them open you may be able to eat them.

Meats that are unprocessed and that do not contain antibiotics are okay. Some examples are beef (lean cuts only), chicken (preferably without the skin), eggs, any fresh or frozen fish that has not been breaded, lamb, pork (lean cuts only), seafood, turkey, and veal. If your health food store doesn't carry antibiotic-free meat (organic meat), ask the butcher at your local supermarket if he or she can order special meats for you. Some supermarket chains have started carrying antibiotic-free meat, so check with the local stores or food co-ops in your area.

Nuts, such as almonds, brazil nuts, cashews, filberts, pecans, and walnuts, are allowed, but you should either shell them yourself or buy them from a health food store to avoid harmful additives. Roasted, salted, and honey-coated nuts should not be eaten.

Make sure the **oils** you buy are unrefined, cold-pressed, and preferably from a health food store. Permitted oils are corn, linseed, olive, safflower, sunflower, soy, and walnut. Olive oil is the best oil to cook foods in and is great as a salad dressing. Fish oils are also acceptable.

Olives are permitted, but check the label to make sure they are additive-free.

Pasta products, including lasagna, macaroni, noodles, pasta shells, spaghetti, and all others that have been made from either whole wheat or vegetable products, are allowed. Other possibilities are two types of Japanese noodles: Kuzu-Kiri, made of corn, and soba noodles, which are made of buckwheat. If you are allergic to wheat, Bifun noodles are wheat-free.

Popcorn, popped without oil and eaten without butter or any other seasonings or additives, is a great snack food and can be eaten as a breakfast cereal. Microwave popcorn is not acceptable because of the many flavor and color additives.

Rice cakes are permitted if they are made of brown rice.

Seeds, such as poppy, pumpkin, sesame, and sunflower, are permitted if your digestive system can tolerate them. Be sure to buy them without additives and preferably at a health food store.

Two **thickeners** for sauces and gravies are arrowroot powder and cornstarch. Specific thickener information is included under the "Cooking Tips" section later in this chapter.

Tofu (bean curd) is a health food that can be purchased fresh at your local food store.

Tomatoes are permitted, but they should be fresh and carefully washed to remove all mold. Canned tomatoes contain added ingredients, including sweeteners. Tomato pastes and sauces are acceptable if they do not contain additives, such as citric acid or sweeteners. The majority do, however, so read the label.

Vegetables are an extremely important part of the diet, but even they should be monitored during stage one. Fresh or frozen vegetables are fine for most patients, although some have found recovery possible only after they limited their diet to organically grown vegetables. Before eating vegetables, be sure to thoroughly scrub them to remove all mold.

Since you must limit your carbohydrates sharply during this stage, vegetables should be broken down into two categories: low-carbohydrate vegetables and high-carbohydrate vegetables. For the first two or three weeks of the diet, limit your intake of the following high-carbohydrate vegetables: beans (dried or cooked), corn, lima beans, peas (dried or cooked), potatoes, and squash (acorn, butternut, or winter). The following vegetables are low in carbohydrates and can be eaten during any stage: asparagus, beets, broccoli, brussels sprouts, cabbage, carrots, cauliflower, celery, cucumbers, eggplant, green peppers, lettuce (all varieties), okra, onions, parsley, radishes, soybeans, string beans, tomatoes (fresh, not canned), and turnips.

Wheatless flours, such as arrowroot, amaranth, buckwheat, corn, millet, rice, potato, spelt, and soy, are good if you are allergic to wheat.

Whole grains, such as barley, corn, flaxseed, millet, oats and oatmeal (not instant), brown rice or wild rice (*not* white rice), rye, and wheat, are allowed but may have to be eaten in moderation. Grains that contain gluten (wheat, rye, barley, and oats) can cause digestive symptoms, so you may want to try healthy and delicious grain alternatives instead, such as buckwheat, teff, quinoa (pronounced keen' wa), and amaranth.

Foods for Stage Two and after the Diet

During stage two, be sure you continue to eat foods high in complex carbohydrates. A diet high in complex carbohydrates promotes health because carbohydrates feed the lactobacilli, and they in turn help keep Candida growth under control. In addition, foods that are high in complex carbohydrates, like grains and vegetables, do not encourage yeast growth because they are digested slowly and can't be broken down to the point where yeasts can ferment them.

Because of their nutrient value, slowly try adding whole fruits to your diet during stage two. Dr. Crook recommends that you eat a small amount of banana (a low-sugar fruit), wait ten minutes, and have a second bite. If you don't have a negative reaction, eat the whole banana. If your body successfully tolerates the banana, try slowly adding another small dose of fruit, such as a strawberry, pineapple, or a tart apple such as a Granny Smith. Remember to add new foods to your diet very slowly and be careful not to overtax your body or overestimate your improved health.

During this stage, you can begin to add a variety of foods to your diet. The first list below includes nutritious foods that will nourish your body and help you on your way to recovery. However, you should eat even these foods in moderation. And remember to add them to your diet gradually to allow your body time to adjust to the change and to watch for sensitivities. The second list includes foods that won't help you recover, but that may be eaten very occasionally if you want them and if your body can tolerate them.

HEALTHY FOODS YOU SHOULD EAT

The following foods are acceptable during stage two and will provide you with valuable nutrients:

Cereals may be added to your diet during stage two, but try to limit those that contain sugar, fruit, flavorings, or malt.

Fruits, in either whole, juice, or dried form, should be added with caution because they contain fructose, a simple sugar that increases Candida growth.

Soured milk products contain vitamins your body needs. Yogurt that does not contain sugar, fruit, or flavorings and that is either made at home or purchased at a health food store is the best choice.

NOT-SO-HEALTHY FOODS YOU MAY BE ABLE TO TOLERATE

There are other foods that are not as healthy or as necessary to your recovery. It would be best if you didn't eat them at all, but they can be eaten occasionally during stage two and after the diet if you are strong enough and don't have allergic reactions to them. Such food choices include the following:

Condiments: Most condiments contain monosodium glutamate, sugar, vinegar, or yeast, so they may have to be avoided. Whether or not you will be able to add condiments during stage two or even after finishing the diet depends on how strong your health is.

Cheeses may be okay, though you should avoid any that contain mold or citric acid.

Flavorings often used in dessert recipes such as vanilla extract, mint extract, and lemon extract often contain alcohol. Check with your health food store to see if or could order flavorings without alcohol or additives.

Fried foods should be avoided but can be eaten occasionally, your health permitting, after you recover.

Leftovers stored in the refrigerator can contain mold. The best alternative is to freeze food.

Margarine should usually be avoided because it contains preservatives, flavorings, and chemical additives.

Meats that have been dried, smoked, or otherwise processed may be eaten occasionally.

Milk should usually be declined in favor of other dairy products because it commonly causes allergic reactions and because it contains lactose, another name for milk sugar. Milk can also contain trace amounts of up to eighty different antibiotics.

Oils not listed in the acceptable foods list are not recommended, including any vegetable oils and coconut, corn, cottonseed, and peanut oils.

Peanuts, peanut products, and pistachios should generally be avoided because they frequently contain mold and fungi.

Spices, which are prone to mold, should be all but excluded from your diet, including regular table salt, which contains additives. Some patients can tolerate spices if they have been cooked along with a meal because the mold would have been destroyed during the cooking process.

Many CRC patients find black pepper hard to digest but cayenne pepper does not seem to cause digestive problems. Cream of tartar (which is technically potassium bitartrate, a chemical used in laxatives and in the tinning of metals) is a spice frequently used in breads, cakes, candies, frostings, and meringues and should be avoided. It is made from the residue in wine barrels and, because of its close association with the fermentation process, can provoke allergic symptoms.

Sweeteners, such as sugar and all sugar products, are forbidden. However, a variety of sweeteners that are less processed and more nutritional than white sugar can be had occasionally when you are done with the diet. These include aguamiel (from maguey cactus and similar to molasses), amazake (from rice), barley malt, beet sugar, brown sugar, honey, molasses, rice syrup, and maple syrup.

Two other sweeteners that are great for recipes are 100 percent pure vegetable glycerine (made from coconut oil), and a healthy sweetener called fructo-oligo-saccharide (FOS), which is widely used in Japan. FOS actually seems to help CRC patients because it inhibits Candida in the body. FOS has been scientifically studied and was found to be safe for consumption.

In *The Woman and the Yeast Connection* Dr. Crook gives a detailed description of FOS and its health benefits. FOS, which is basically sucrose with additionally attached fructose molecules, appears naturally in vegetables, grains, and some fruits. However, some side effects have been reported—mostly digestive problems such as gas, abdominal pain, and diarrhea.

FOS is not absorbed in the GI tract, and it actually increases growth of lactobacilli and bifidus, two of the friendly bacteria in your body that fight Candida. FOS is expensive, however. It costs about $10 to $12 for one hundred grams or one-half a cup. It is very concentrated, though, so a little goes a long way. If you decide to try FOS, start by adding it slowly to your diet.

Foods to Be Avoided Even after the Diet
In general, you will need to avoid poor quality foods, including processed, packaged, and junk foods, all of which contain hidden ingredients (including salt and sugar) and are likely to have low nutrient value. Junk food is refined and overly processed and often contains ingredients such as sugar, salt, food coloring, additives, and vegetable oil. White flour and sugar, two highly refined foods, contain the refined carbohydrates that increase Candida growth.

Although refined foods are obviously bad because they lack nutrients, contain additives, and are in general unhealthy, there is another reason they should be avoided. In *Back to Health*, Dr. Remington explains that as defense mechanisms against the fungi around them, many plants contain natural antifungal structures or chemical substances. When foods are refined, the natural chemicals are removed. Dr. Remington cites the example of wheat, which has an antifungal outer layer designed to naturally protect the plant as it grows. When wheat is milled the outer layer is removed.

Many of the foods listed in this section contain harmful additives such as colorings, preservatives, and sugars. For example, two additives that are specifically derived from yeast and will therefore cause symptoms are citric acid and monosodium glutamate.

The following is a list of foods and products you should avoid during and after the Candida control diet.

Alcoholic and fermented beverages, including cider and root beer, must be avoided because they contain yeast and often sugar.

Beverages, such as soda, coffee, and tea, including herb teas (because they can contain mold), have to be omitted from your diet.

Caffeine, or anything that contains caffeine, must be strictly avoided.

Fungi, such as mushrooms, morels, and truffles, have to be avoided because, like mold, they cause allergic reactions.

Malt and malt products such as candy, cereals, and malted drinks should be eaten only rarely.

Packaged and processed foods, such as cake mixes, cheese and macaroni, or anything in a box that basically lacks nutrient value, should be avoided.

Sugar must be absolutely avoided, especially simple carbohydrate sugars such as cane sugar, honey (which also contains yeast spores), molasses, maple syrup, maple sugar, date sugar, and turbinado sugar. Whenever possible avoid artificial sweeteners such as NutraSweet (aspartame) because of their chemical nature. Before you buy foods at the store carefully read the labels to make sure they do not contain these forms of sugar: dextrose, fructose, galactose, glucose, glycogen, lactose, maltose, mannitol, monosaccharides, NutraSweet, polysaccharides, sorbitol, and sucrose.

Vinegar and vinegar-containing foods such as mayonnaise, mustard, pickles, salad dressing, sauerkraut, soy sauce, and tamari must be avoided because they contain yeast.

White flour and refined grain products such as pasta made from white flour must be avoided because of their low nutrient value. You may find after completing the diet that you can tolerate small amounts of refined products such as white flour.

Because CRC affects patients in different ways and some cases are more severe than others, there are no exact rules about what to eat after your CRC is under control. A diet high in sugar and lacking in nutrients will keep you from recovering from CRC, and a similar diet afterward can only hurt your health. For best results, continue to rotate your foods, avoid foods you crave or are allergic to, and avoid processed foods and those included in last list above.

Several CRC cookbooks with extensive dietary information are available, and their nutritious and delicious recipes will simplify your life. Although there are many cookbooks available, three of the most helpful and easy-to-read are the following:

- *The Candida Control Cookbook* by Gail Burton. A gourmet cook, former food columnist, and CRC patient herself, Burton provides helpful dietary advice. Her recipes are simple but delicious. An excellent book overall.
- *The Yeast Connection Cookbook: A Guide to Good Nutrition and Better Health* by William G. Crook, M.D., and Marjorie Hurt Jones, R.N. This cookbook provides comprehensive dietary information and a wide range of recipes for every aspect of the diet.
- *The Candida Directory and Cookbook* by Helen Gustafson and Maureen O'Shea. This team of authors, one a CRC patient and the other a nutritional counselor, provides us with unique and tasty recipes from a variety of cooks, including Julia Child.

Living on the Candida Control Diet

While dietary recommendations and acceptable food are important parts of the diet, living with the diet involves more than lists and guidelines. Finding the foods you need both in the grocery store and in restaurants may initially be a challenge.

Breakfast: Your Daily Wake-Up Call

The staples of a regular American breakfast, which include bread or bread items, fruit juices, milk, coffee, tea, and processed meats, are forbidden during stage one of the diet. This doesn't mean, however, that finding an acceptable, nutritious, fast, and easy meal will be difficult or even time-consuming. A wide variety of breakfast foods are permitted as part of the diet, but don't forget to rotate your foods (have one item every four to seven days) so as not to become allergic or addicted to frequently eaten foods.

Perhaps the most important breakfast tip is to either prepare your breakfast the day before or go to bed thinking about tomorrow's early morning meal. Although the temptation to skip this meal might be great, breakfast really is the most important meal of the day, and getting enough nutrition is crucial to your recovery. Remember, your recovery depends on your ability to take care of yourself, and neglecting to prepare nutritious breakfasts will only delay it.

Some breakfast suggestions include the following items, but don't be afraid to experiment with quick and easy alternatives. You can save time by making large batches of food and freezing them for later. Most of these suggestions fit into stage two of the diet.

- Biscuits, breads, flatbread, French toast, muffins, pancakes, popovers, or waffles can be made from an acceptable grain or grain alternative.

- Brown rice as a side dish to eggs or a bread item is quick and nutritious.
- A wide variety of cereals are available at grocery and health food stores, but make sure they aren't processed and that they don't contain additives, yeast, sugar, or malt. Perhaps the most nutritious and certain additive-free cereals are the ones you make yourself. Some store-bought cereals you may be able to eat are cracked wheat, cream of brown rice, cream of rye, cream of wheat, grits, oat bran, oatmeal (but not instant), puffed corn, puffed millet, puffed rice, puffed wheat, shredded wheat, shredded wheat and bran, Wheatena, wheat hearts, and Zoom. You should also be able to tolerate cereals sweetened with fruit juice.
- Healthy crackers spread with tahini or hummus are an easy and fast meal.
- Eggs can be hard-boiled, scrambled, poached, or served as an frittata, omelet, or soufflé.
- A grapefruit and melon are options, but be sure to thoroughly wash them because they can contain mold.
- Potatoes, or other vegetables, are often relegated to the lunch or dinner menu and overlooked as a breakfast food. Carrots, celery, or any other vegetables can be eaten raw, shredded, or diced.
- Rice cakes with a nut or other tasty butter are a quick and healthy breakfast.

In her book *Silent Menace: Twentieth Century Epidemic—Candidiasis*, Dorothy Senerchia, a CRC patient herself, offers a list of breakfast suggestions for people following the Candida control diet:

- Guacamole with yeast-free crackers.
- Lentil or vegetable soup.
- Homemade gelatin (additive-free and from your health food store) made with a small amount of fresh fruit juice (when you can tolerate it).
- Rice pudding made from either brown or white rice.
- Soken's vegetable chips spread with sunflower, sesame, or almond butter.
- Soybean or tofu milkshake made with fruit or fruit juice (save this for when you can tolerate fruit). Use one or more of the following fruits: peach, nectarine, pear, mango, or banana.

Breakfast doesn't have to be boring, repetitious, or even difficult when you consider the variety of food you have to choose from. As your health improves, you may be able to add processed meats and small amounts of fruit to liven up your first meal of the day.

Cooking Tips

Since refined, packaged, and processed foods are not allowed on the Candida control diet, you may find yourself cooking quite a bit. Although cookbooks designed for CRC patients are your best bet, this sections offers some simple recipes and cooking tips.

In *The Candida Control Cookbook,* Gail Burton provides an easy recipe for clarified butter, which is a healthier version of butter because it removes the milk sugar. Burton suggests clarifying a large amount of butter at one time and storing it for later use. The recipe calls for one half-cup to one pound of unsalted butter. To prepare on a stove, heat the butter in a small skillet. After the butter has melted and completely separated into a white substance and clear yellow liquid, discard the white substance and pour the yellow liquid into a storage container. Throw away any residue at the bottom of the pan. After your clarified butter has cooled, seal the container with a lid and store in your refrigerator. You can also clarify butter using your microwave oven: the only change involves heating the butter in a different manner. Cut the butter into one-quarter-inch squares and heat at a medium-high temperature for several seconds.

Because it contains lactose (milk sugar) and trace amounts of antibiotics, milk should be avoided. While limiting the amount of milk you drink may not be difficult, milk is frequently called for in recipes. Providing a substitution is crucial because milk is sometimes the only liquid in recipes other than eggs. Three possible milk substitutes are soy milk, nut milk, and egg whites. Consult a CRC cookbook for information on how to make soy milk and nut milk. To determine how many egg whites to add to your recipe in place of milk use this simple formula: one large egg white equals about three-fourths to one cup of milk. To prepare egg whites, beat them until they are creamy and add as you would milk.

An easy recipe for a nutritious nut spread is to blend one-half cup of either raw almonds, pecans, or walnuts with one tablespoon safflower oil. This nut spread can be used to liven up rice cakes, crackers, biscuits, or just about anything.

In *Silent Menace*, Dorothy Senerchia offers a handy flour substitution chart to help those patients who cannot tolerate wheat develop wheat-free recipes. When baking, don't hesitate to experiment or to be creative.

One cup of wheat flour is equal to:

- One cup millet meal
- One and 1/4 cups rye flour
- One cup corn flour
- 3/4 cup coarse cornmeal
- 3/4 cup plus two tablespoons brown or white rice flour
- 7/8 cup buckwheat flour
- 7/8 cup amaranth flour
- One and 1/3 cups soybean flour
- One and 1/3 cups oat flour or rolled oats
- 1/2 cup barley flour
- 1/2 cup arrowroot flour (starch)
- 1/2 cup plus two tablespoons potato starch (flour)

In her book, Senerchia also gives information on thickener equivalents and a corn-free baking powder for people who are allergic to corn. According to Senerchia, when looking for a thickener for recipes, the following measurements are equal to two tablespoons of wheat flour.

- One tablespoon arrowroot powder (starch or flour)
- One tablespoon potato starch (flour)
- One tablespoon cornstarch
- One tablespoon sweet rice flour
- Two tablespoons millet meal
- Two tablespoons quick-cooking tapioca

Patients allergic to corn may want to try this recipe for corn-free baking powder. To prepare the baking powder, mix three tablespoons of the following ingredients: cream of tartar, arrowroot powder, and baking soda. Potato starch can be used instead of arrowroot powder. After mixing, store tightly covered in a dark place and use as you would any other baking powder. The shelf life of corn-free baking powder is about two to three months, so be sure to write the date on each new batch. If you use this recipe, be careful. Because cream of tartar is closely linked with the fermentation process, some people might be allergic to it, especially during stage one of the diet.

Getting the Foods You Need: Advice on Grocery Shopping

Grocery shopping doesn't have to be difficult or even time-consuming once you develop an easy-to-follow pattern, which includes determining which stores carry your items.

It is extremely important that you buy the purest foods and most unprocessed foods as often as possible. Be sure to buy fruit and vegetables that appear fresh and mold-free. It is also a good idea to buy them from a reputable source. For best results, organically grown produce is highly recommended, especially for chemically sensitive patients. The best way to obtain organically grown vegetables in your area is to contact local farmers. See if they raise their produce organically, and either buy produce at a farmer's market or get some friends together and start a co-op.

Unfortunately, foods that do not contain harmful ingredients usually cost more money. In regular grocery stores these foods are considered specialty items, and the stores charge higher prices. In general, the foods found in health food stores also tend to be more expensive than foods in large supermarkets. You may not want to spend the extra money to buy the more expensive food items, but consider the importance the Candida control diet and proper nutrition play in helping you regain your health. Without proper nutrition, your chances of recovering from CRC drastically decrease; your health will not be regained in large steps, but in small ones.

To avoid additives while you increase the nutrient content of your foods and save money, try preparing foods yourself instead of buying them. Some examples of foods you can prepare yourself are milk substitutes, salad dressings, mayonnaise, rolls, breads, nut spreads or butters, clarified butter, or any other foods that contain few ingredients.

Other helpful grocery shopping hints follow:

- In regular supermarkets, the whole and less-processed foods you can eat are located on the outer walls of the store. If possible, try to avoid the inner aisles, which usually contain packaged and non-nutritious foods.

- Read *everything* on every label, front and back, even on products advertised as sugar-free (this usually just means they lack refined table sugar) and preservative-free. When in doubt, don't buy it.

- Make comprehensive shopping lists and plan your meals ahead of time.

- See if any grocery or health food stores deliver (explain your situation).

- Find a store to order organic meats for you.

- Avoid canned foods because of the high number of additives.

- To add some variety to your diet, try fruits and vegetables you have never heard of before, such as boniata (a sweet type of potato), chayote (a squashlike fruit), daikon (also called an oriental radish), and jicama (similar to a turnip).

Traveling and Socializing on the Diet

Being away from your kitchen doesn't mean you have to refrain from eating or settle for less-than-perfect food. The best way to ensure that nutritious and healthy food will be at your fingertips is to bring your food with you. Bringing your snacks and meals will not only save you time and money, but also guarantee the purity and availability of your food.

Dorothy Senerchia suggests that patients assemble a "survival kit," which can be used while traveling or socializing at parties. The following lists can also be used as possible suggestions for packing your lunch everyday. As your health improves, try adding foods from the stage two list. Here are some of the ingredients of Senerchia's survival kit, a great help for eating on the go:

Utensils	Stage One Foods	Stage Two Foods
can opener	raw vegetables	cheeses
paper napkins	hard-boiled egg	fruit
paper plates	yeast-free crackers	fruit juices
small plastic bag for garbage	rice cakes	can of tuna
plastic silverware	nuts and seeds	can of salmon
small paring knife	nut and seed spreads	can of sardines
	safe potato chips	celery with cheese
	safe tortilla chips	celery with nut spread
	brown rice chips	yogurt dip with crackers
	cold chicken	cream cheese
	stir-fried dish	fresh goat cheese dip
	homemade meat loaf	tofu-avocado dip
	cold shrimp, with homemade mayo	herb tea bags
	homemade soup (in a thermos)	iced herb tea (in a thermos)
	sliced turkey	
	sliced roast beef	
	vegetable salad with lemon and oil dressing	
	black olives (American and not cured)	
	guacamole with yeast-free crackers	

As with breakfast, it is important to plan ahead, be creative, and most importantly, not skip the meals you need to regain your health.

The Ins and Outs of Dining Out

Whether or not you can eat out depends on how severely your Candida is affecting you. Patients with severe cases report that they can find nothing tolerable in restaurants. Other patients find that if they stick to grilled vegetables and skip dessert they are all right. As is to be expected, when dining out keep three considerations in mind: what types of foods you are eating, the ingredients in those types of foods, and at what type of restaurant you are eating.

Some suggestions for selecting foods in a restaurant are below:

- Stick to basic, plain foods (such as meats and vegetables).
- Order foods you are in the habit of eating, such as chicken or a salad.
- Avoid all mushrooms, sauces, and gravies.
- Safe beverage choices are bottled water, soda water, sparkling water, or mineral water.

Gail Burton offers these handy tips:

- Skip the bread basket.
- Avoid entreés cooked with flour, milk, sugar, or wine, but ones cooked with butter, lemon, or olive oil are acceptable.
- Have lemon with your shrimp cocktail instead of sauce.
- Don't have sour cream with your baked potato.

Be sure to pick restaurants likely to accommodate your special dietary needs. The safest way to find out is to call ahead of time and briefly explain your dietary restrictions. Don't be afraid to ask pointed questions about the ingredients of the meals you are interested in and/or ask for changes or substitutions. In *The Candida Cookbook and Directory*, Gustafson and O'Shea recommend Chinese and Iranian restaurants as the safest places to eat. "Chinese cooks are wonderful about making dishes to order and Iranians are strong on naturally whole foods like rice and vegetables along with plain, grilled shish-kabob. They often include grilled eggplant and peppers."

Because of their style, traditional French restaurants aren't recommended for CRC patients. French cuisine, with its heavy sauces and seasonings, contains ingredients that are likely to cause allergic reactions. Because of their traditional foods, Chinese, Greek, Italian, and Mexican restaurants are acceptable, although you should still investigate individual restaurants and dishes.

As expected, fast food restaurants provide few foods for CRC patients. If you have to eat at one, your best bet is to get a salad without dressing. As for American restaurants, try to order plain meat or fish (no sauce), a salad without dressing, and simple grilled or steamed vegetables flavored with only butter.

If you are sensitive to all foods but the ones you prepare yourself, remember that there are other ways to spend time and have fun with your friends and family. As Dorothy Senerchia writes, "It's also important to consider that not all your social activities have to be centered around food and drink. With the same people you might ordinarily meet for a meal, you can take a walk in a park, go to the health club, take a drive in the country, or plan some other entertainment. Movies, for example, have no yeast."

Living with CRC doesn't mean eating boring and tasteless food for the rest of your life: it means you are serious about and value your health. By following the Candida control diet you are taking a big step toward controlling CRC and changing the way you live. Once you have abandoned foods loaded with sugar, salt, preservatives, additives, and other harmful poisons, you will probably never be able to return to them again. There are two reasons for this: your tastes will have changed, and you will never be able to look at food and your health in the same manner again. You will still be able to enjoy good food and savory dishes, but you will choose foods that enhance your health instead of harm it.

—10—

Prescription Medications

Formerly, when religion was strong and science weak, men mistook magic for medicine; now, when science is strong and religion weak, men mistake medicine for magic.
—Thomas Szasz in *The Second Sin*

For the majority of patients, antifungal medications in combination with the Candida control diet can help get CRC under control. The medications described in this chapter cannot cure CRC, but can help you recover by killing large amounts of Candida organisms. Remember, the symptoms of CRC are caused by the Candida organism, but the real problem is the weakened immune system that allowed the Candida organism to grow out of control. Reducing the amount of Candida in the body is crucial to recovery since Candida overgrowth further suppresses the immune system. By killing large amounts of Candida, medications reduce the suppression of the immune system, which then helps restore your own immune defenses.

Some patients prefer not to take antifungal medicines because other medications caused their CRC, and they would rather try to recover from Candida by taking *Lactobacillus acidophilus* and other natural remedies. However, patients with severe cases of CRC should seriously consider taking antifungal medicines so as not to prolong their illness.

It is extremely important to work with your physician when selecting the medications you will need to overcome CRC. A drug selected for a friend or family member may be inappropriate or unsafe for you, and the side effects of drugs can vary from person to

121

person. Your physician takes three factors into account when he or she prescribes a medication for you: the particular characteristics or needs of you as a patient; how the illness, in this case CRC, is manifesting itself in your particular case; and the experiences and comfort level he has with the medications used to treat CRC.

Although the following section gives the latest information on the drugs commonly used to treat CRC, a physician should be both your guide to proper use and your source for the most recent drug information. Anytime you work with your physician, it is important to let him know of your interest in your health care and your intent to participate fully and equally.

If you have any questions as to why your doctor has chosen a particular medication for you, be sure to ask. Because each case of CRC differs from every other case, your physician may not be able to give you exact answers. However, asking questions gives voice to your concerns and shows your intent to participate in the struggle to regain your health. It is important you begin to be an *activated patient* (a term made popular by Dr. Sehnert) and that you establish an open and equal relationship with your doctor. Some questions you may want to ask follow:

- What effects should I expect from this medication?
- Is there any chance I could become addicted or dependent on this drug?
- How long will I have to take this medication?
- What will be our next step if the medication doesn't help me?
- Is there a wide gap between the therapeutic and toxic amounts of this drug?
- What if I become pregnant while taking this drug?

As a patient, your responsibilities include the following:

- Reporting to your physician any side effects or changes in your body, even if they seem trivial or are embarrassing.
- Not changing the dosage amount or schedule without your doctor's explicit permission.

Correctly using any medication involves two types of knowledge: specific knowledge of the drug or family of drugs involved, and a general understanding of how to use medications. This chapter provides specific information on how to work with your doctor in order to ensure that you use your medications correctly, and specific knowledge of the antifungal drugs commonly prescribed for CRC. Using your medications safely involves two extremely important features: common sense and caution. As long as you are in constant communication with your physician and you are sensible and careful with the usage of your medications (both over-the-counter and prescription), few problems relating to medication usage should occur.

Prescription Antifungal Drugs: Powerful Tools in the War against Candida

Simply defined, antifungal drugs stop or prevent the growth of fungi, in this case Candida. There are two types of prescription antifungal drugs commonly used to treat CRC: one set is nystatin and amphotericin B, and the other set is a family of drugs called the azoles. One marked difference between the two groups is that one is hardly absorbed into the bloodstream, while the other is largely absorbed into the bloodstream.

The drugs that are, for the most part, not absorbed into the bloodstream include nystatin USP, either powder or tablets. Brand names of nystatin are Nilstat, Nystex, and Mycostatin. Another drug that isn't absorbed into the bloodstream is amphotericin B, the brand name of which is Fungizone Intravenous. The drugs which are absorbed into the bloodstream are the azole family of antifungal drugs, fluconazole (brand name Diflucan), ketoconazole (brand name Nizerol), and itraconazole (brand name Sporanox). Although the information below pertains to the systemic forms of the five antifungal drugs used to treat CRC, all are also available in topical versions, such as ointments and creams, some of which can be used to treat fungal infections of the skin.

The information below is designed to help you understand four things: the drugs themselves, how these drugs work, the role of the drug in treating CRC, and general information outlining which drugs are more appropriate for which people and which situations. This information should not replace your physician's advice or counsel, since she is most familiar with your personal health needs and medical history. Your doctor is your final source for the latest information on these drugs and whether or not their use is appropriate for you.

The Azoles

The azole family of drugs is made up of extremely effective antifungal medicines that are constructed of synthetic compounds. Before the introduction of the azole drugs (starting with Nizerol in 1981 and followed by the other two in the 1990s), intravenous amphotericin B, which came out in the late 1950s, was the standard treatment for deep-seated fungal infections. According to a 1994 article in the *New England Journal of Medicine (NEJM)*, "The oral azole drugs—ketoconazole, fluconazole, and itraconazole—represent a major advance in systemic antifungal therapy."

In summing up its comparison of the three drugs, the *NEJM* came to two conclusions. It decided fluconazole (Diflucan) has the most attractive pharmacologic profile. Ketoconazole (Nizerol), on the other hand, is the least tolerated by patients and has the most toxic effects. However, it is also the least expensive of the three drugs, which is an important factor when you consider many patients require long-term therapy. The *NEJM* article also concluded that the three drugs are effective alternatives to intravenous amphotericin B therapy.

Azoles inhibit fungi by attacking a component of the fungal cell membrane. Since they are systemic, which means the medication travels throughout the body, there are greater chances of toxicity and side effects than when amphotericin B and nystatin are used, although the overall chances for side effects remain small. Still, because of this increased chance of side effects, some doctors reserve the azoles for patients who are not responding to nystatin, even though they have had fairly positive results with most or all three azole drugs.

It is important to note that patients who are allergic to one azole may be allergic to the other azoles. Be sure to discuss any medical problems you may have and your medical history with your physician. Be especially sure to tell him or her if you have achlorhydria, which is the absence of stomach acid, or hypochlorhydria, which is decreased stomach acid, because these problems may affect the use of azoles. It is also crucial to mention whether or not you presently abuse alcohol, or if you have a history of alcohol abuse, or if you have liver or kidney disease.

As with all medications, be sure to tell your physician if you are taking any other nonprescription or prescription medications. Check with your physician before taking any other medications while you are still taking antifungal medications. Never take Seldane or Hismanal while taking an azole. Serious heart problems or even death could occur. Certain conditions that should be met regarding the use of azoles include the following:

- Take this medication for the full prescribed time of treatment, even if you feel better or your symptoms disappear. Because fungal illnesses are difficult to treat and take a long time to clear out of the body, it is very important to continue taking your medication for the specific length of time your physician recommends.

- Be careful not to miss any doses because the azole drugs are most effective when there is a constant amount in the blood. It is also important to take each dose at the same time every day. If you do miss a dose, take it as soon as possible. If too much time has elapsed, just skip the missed dose and wait for your next scheduled dose. If you miss a dose, do not double your next dose.
- Avoid all alcoholic beverages while taking azoles, including alcohol-containing preparations, such as over-the-counter elixirs, cough syrups, and tonics. The use of alcoholic beverages increases the chances of liver problems and can cause stomach pain, vomiting, nausea, and other problems. It is also a good idea to avoid alcohol for one day after stopping azoles to give the body time to fully rid itself of the medication.
- Avoid antacids, which should not be taken when you are on any of the azole medications. Do not take Tagamet, Zantac, or other similar medications either.
- Take Nizerol and Sporanox with a meal or snack.

Although the following symptoms are uncommon, if you develop them while taking azole medications, seek medical attention. Symptoms include skin rashes or itching, fever with chills, loss of appetite, changes in your skin or mucous membranes, stomach pain, yellow eyes or skin, and unusual tiredness or weakness. If your symptoms do not improve after several weeks, or if your symptoms worsen, see your doctor immediately. When taking azoles, it is important that you have regular visits with your physician so she can monitor your progress and check for negative side effects.

Below is a description and discussion of the three different azole drugs, including their individual benefits and drawbacks.

Nizerol (Ketoconazole): Unlike nystatin, Nizerol is absorbed into the bloodstream. This is both an advantage and disadvantage over nystatin. Physicians often prescribe Nizerol when nystatin and other medications do not work. However, some physicians prefer Nizerol to nystatin. Dr. Crook quotes Allan Lieberman, M.D., of South Carolina as saying that it is his medication of choice because it provides a more dramatic improvement and acts more promptly than nystatin. Nizerol also produces less die-off reactions than nystatin. Lieberman reported that he has treated hundreds of patients with Nizerol and none has ever experienced a severe reaction. Based on his experiences, he concluded Nizerol is an extremely useful drug.

The best known and most serious side effect of Nizerol is possible liver problems, although only one in ten thousand patients who took it had inflammation of the liver or other serious adverse reactions. According to the 1995 *USP DI Advice for the Health Care Professional*, "It [hepatotoxicity] is usually, but not always, reversible upon discontinuation of ketoconazole, and fatalities have been reported rarely. It is considered to be an idiosyncratic [peculiar to an individual] reaction and can occur at any time during therapy." Symptoms of possible liver problems or damage include unusual fatigue, nausea or vomiting, loss of appetite, dark urine, or pale stools. Because of the possible liver problems, blood tests to monitor liver function need to be performed every month and more often if the daily dose exceeds one tablet, which is 200 mg.

Nizerol is also known to sometimes cause drowsiness and dizziness in some people. Two other side effects of this azole are heightened sensitivity of patients' eyes to light and possible endocrine dysfunction, which can include menstrual irregularities, enlarged breasts in the male, deficient sperm production, loss of libido, and impotence.

Diflucan (Fluconazole): Diflucan, a cousin of Nizerol, was approved for use in the United States in 1990. In his book, *Candida*, Luc De Schepper, M.D., writes, "With the appearance of Diflucan, all the other antifungal medications have taken a back seat. In a study done by the Division of Infectious Diseases, at St. Pierre University Hospital, Brussels, Belgium, the efficacy of Diflucan was compared with Nizerol and found to be twice as effective and much less toxic for the liver."

Diflucan is widely distributed throughout the body and absorbed more completely into the tissues than Nizerol. Many physicians prefer it to Nizerol because of Nizerol's possible liver side effects, and some report that Diflucan works better for their patients who have skin problems. Overall, however, Diflucan appears to be safer, better tolerated by patients, and more effective than Nizerol. One drawback of Diflucan is the high cost of about $7 per pill.

Side effects appear to be minimal (mostly gastrointestinal disturbances), and no toxic effects have been reported. Although no liver problems have been associated with Diflucan, the manufacturers recommend a liver function test one month after taking it. Dr. Remington, a practicing physician, performs a routine liver enzyme test even though this medication appears to have less potential for liver problems.

Sporanox (Itraconazole): Although Sporanox, like Diflucan, is new on the market, physicians and patients have found it to be safe and effective. Sporanox, another azole, was licensed for use in 1993.

In a 1989 article published in *Drugs*, Susan M. Grant and S. P. Clissold highlighted the positive and negative features of Sporanox.

They concluded that it was highly effective and that generally greater than 80 percent of patients with superficial skin problems or yeast infections were "cured" or markedly improved after it. They also found Sporanox to be well tolerated by most patients, with the most common side effects relating to gastrointestinal disturbances.

Another article noted that of the fifteen thousand patients treated with Sporanox, only 7 percent experienced side effects, and gastrointestinal problems and headaches were the most frequent complaints. This article also cites the 80 percent cure rate and adds that Sporanox has been distributed in forty-eight countries.

Nystatin and Amphotericin B

Nilstat, Nystex, or Mycostatin (Nystatin, USP): Many physicians specifically prescribe nystatin instead of the other antifungal drugs available because it is inexpensive, safe, and effective. Doctors frequently prescribe nystatin first for their patients, and if it doesn't work they then try the azole drugs.

Nystatin was first discovered in 1950 and has a wide range of antifungal activity. Dr. Truss said he personally prefers to prescribe nystatin, as does Dr. Sehnert. Dr. Truss described nystatin as being a topical drug that has been on the market for over four decades without toxicity. "It is as close to perfect as you could design," he said.

Dr. Crook also prefers nystatin and writes in *The Yeast Connection* that "nystatin is the medication I usually prescribe for my patients with yeast-connected health problems." He also stressed the safety of using nystatin, which is supported by the *Physician's Desk Reference* (*PDR*), a major source of drug information for physicians. Dr. Crook said that while he did not make a page-by-page search of the *PDR*, he was able to conclude that "nystatin was easily the safest of all prescription medications."

Nystatin is available in many forms: chemically pure powder, pill, liquid oral suspension, vaginal tablets and suppositories, and topical powders. The liquid oral suspension, which is commonly given to infants and children, should be avoided because it contains sugar, which increases Candida growth.

Despite the inconvenience of the powdered form, which has to be added to water (although it is insoluble) or dissolved in the mouth, most physicians prefer the powdered form of nystatin because it does not contain excipients, which are inert substances such as fillers, food colorings, or other additives that can cause allergic reactions in sensitive patients. The powdered form is also more economical. It should not be refrigerated, as its potency will decrease.

Many patients find that taking the powdered form of nystatin is inconvenient during the day (at work or while traveling), so they take the powder in the morning and evening and the tablets in the middle of the day. Nystatin damages the Candida cell walls, which results in the destruction of the organisms. The reason nystatin is so safe is because it isn't absorbed into the bloodstream in amounts large enough to cause many side effects or to be a risk to the patient. Research shows that the extremely small amounts of nystatin that are absorbed into the blood are beneficial and help kill Candida throughout the body.

Although most patients have positive impressions of the drug, some patients do have trouble tolerating nystatin and report digestive symptoms, skin rashes, fatigue, and headaches. Even when initial symptoms do occur, they recede when patients continue to take this medication. Since Nystatin kills Candida rather brutally, the die-off effects are generally much worse than with other medications. These also lessen with time. Nystatin is taken in large oral doses because it works in the intestinal and digestive tracts and a lot of medicine is needed to cover the large surface area of these organs. Vaginal tablets and suppositories containing nystatin are also used to relieve the discomfort of vaginal yeast infections.

As with any medication, if you are pregnant, be sure to talk to your physician before taking nystatin. Dr. Remington points out, however, that patients and their unborn children don't seem to suffer any negative effects from taking nystatin during pregnancy:

> Although no problems have been reported from using nystatin during pregnancy, and although the drug contains no warnings, we suggest that you wait until you are past the thirteen-week point in your pregnancy before taking nystatin. If your symptoms are severe, or if you get pregnant while on treatment, you may wish to continue taking the nystatin, but don't exceed one-fourth of a teaspoon (two pills) four times daily. Since very little nystatin is absorbed into the bloodstream, very little—if any—gets into the breast milk, so taking it during breast-feeding appears to be safe. Nystatin is tolerated even in high doses by infants.

Although there are other drugs on the market used to treat CRC, nystatin is considered extremely safe and effective, so it is very likely that your physician will prescribe nystatin for you. Unlike antibiotics, heavy use of which often leads to drug-resistant bacteria, Candida resistance to nystatin seems to happen infrequently. Although nystatin-resistant Candida strains can be produced in laboratories, when it comes to human disease they are rare or nonexistent. A study of two thousand strains of Candida showed no nystatin-resistant strains.

Fungizone and Fungizone Intravenous (Amphotericin B):
Amphotericin B is the leading oral antifungal medication in Europe and comes in three forms: oral, intravenous, and topical. Until very recently, amphotericin B was available only in intravenous form in the United States, and patients who needed the oral form had to order it from France. It is now becoming available in the United States.

There are tremendous differences between the oral and intravenous forms of amphotericin B. Oral amphotericin B is safe and effective, while the intravenous version has serious side effects and is known to be toxic. The oral form of amphotericin B is similar to nystatin in that little of it is absorbed into the bloodstream, and it has a wide range of activity against Candida. Of all the medications available to treat CRC, amphotericin B is perhaps the least often used. Two reasons for this are because of the difficulty involved in obtaining the oral form and because physicians may assume the toxic side effects of the intravenous form of amphotericin B apply to the oral version as well.

If intravenous amphotericin B is so toxic, then why is it even used? According to the 1995 *USP DI Advice for the Health Care Professional*, because intravenous amphotericin B is "frequently the only effective treatment for certain potentially fatal fungal infections, its lifesaving benefits must be balanced against its potential for dangerous side/adverse effects." One very serious side effect is kidney problems. Commonly reported side effects also include fever and chills, headaches, irregular heartbeat, vomiting, and unusual tiredness or weakness. Another reason intravenous amphotericin B could cause problems is because it is capable of negatively interacting with a large amount of other medications. In fact, the 1995 edition of the *USP DI Advice for the Patient: Drug Information in Lay Language* lists not less than thirty-four medicines, types of medicine, families of medicines, or medical procedures (including X-ray treatments) that could cause interactions with intravenous amphotericin B.

The pill form of the drug, however, is considered to be (like nystatin) safe and effective because little is absorbed into the bloodstream. In fact, the *Physician's Desk Reference* (*PDR*) reports that amphotericin B is substantially more effective against Candida than nystatin. As Dr. Crook's comments in *The Yeast Connection* suggest, many physicians who do prescribe oral amphotericin B do so when their patients fail to improve on nystatin:

> These data certainly suggest that oral amphotericin B should be a safe alternative anti-Candida medication—especially for patients who: (1) do not tolerate nystatin, (2) fail to improve on nystatin or (3) relapse when taking nys-

tatin after an initial period of improvement. Between March and August of 1983, a number of patients who did not tolerate or who failed to improve while taking nystatin obtained amphotericin B from France, and several showed an excellent response.

Since amphotericin B is now available in pill form in the U.S. and is an effective treatment for CRC, there is every reason to believe physicians may readily prescribe it for patients who have used nystatin without success. Like the other medications detailed in this chapter, amphotericin B doesn't work for all the patients who take it, but it does work for a significant number. Two pharmacies in the U.S. that now sell oral amphotericin B are Wellness Health & Pharmaceuticals, (800) 227-2627, and College Pharmacy, (800) 888-9358.

Prescription antifungal medications have been used with great success to treat patients with CRC. When used correctly, these medications usually give the body the help it needs to reactivate its own defenses and begin clearing the body of Candida overgrowth.

—11—

Additional Treatments

One of the first duties of the physician is to educate the masses not to take medicine.
—Sir William Osler, quoted by William B. Bean in
Sir William Osler: Aphorisms

Although medications and a careful diet are crucial to recovery from CRC, additional treatments such as *Lactobacillus acidophilus* supplements and a variety of others are equally important. All treatments for CRC have two goals in mind: to reduce the amount of Candida in the body and to boost the immune system. Some suggested treatments include the following:

- treating common CRC symptoms through supplements
- probiotics (friendly bacteria)
- nonprescription antifungal remedies that specifically kill Candida
- substances that naturally boost the immune system
- substances that aid digestion
- proper colon health

This section is not a substitute for the Candida control diet or any of the necessary medications, but rather is intended to complement the therapies already explained in this book.

Treating Common CRC Symptoms with Supplements

The following is a brief inventory of the vitamins, minerals, and other supplements able to reduce or alleviate common CRC symptoms. This listing is by no means comprehensive and cannot replace the advice of your physician. Recovery from CRC is difficult, but if recovery truly is your goal, it is important that you do not simply treat your symptoms, but rather follow the sometimes difficult (but extremely important and necessary) therapies listed in this book.

In general, the vitamins and minerals that seem to alleviate the most CRC symptoms include vitamin B complex, vitamin B_6, magnesium/ calcium (they should always be taken together), vitamin C, coenzyme Q_{10}, and zinc. It is especially important to supplement your diet with both magnesium and vitamin B_6 because both are depleted by Candida overgrowth. Some patients have found that a natural food supplement called Green Magma, made by the Green Foods Corporation, improves their overall health. Green Magma is a pure natural juice made from young barley leaves and brown rice. An excellent source of digestive enzymes, Green Magma also has large concentrations of vitamins, minerals, proteins, chlorophyll, and other nutrients.

Below is a listing of supplements to help alleviate some specific CRC symptoms.

Acne: Nystatin, vitamin A, vitamin B complex, vitamin B_6 (especially for premenstrual or menstrual acne), zinc, and essential fatty acids.

Allergies: Vitamin B_6 and coenzyme Q_{10} (CoQ_{10}).

Anxiety: Vitamin B complex, vitamin B_6, folic acid (which should be taken with vitamin B_{12}), and zinc. Ginkgo biloba extract can help with the emotional instability linked to anxiety. Ginkgo biloba extract comes from the leaves of the Ginkgo trees, which are the oldest living trees on earth and are found in China. In Germany and France, Ginkgo biloba extracts are among the most commonly prescribed drugs and are used to treat heart and eye diseases and brain trauma.

Depression: Vitamin B_6, magnesium, folic acid (which should be taken with vitamin B_{12}), vitamin B complex, Ginkgo biloba, and zinc.

Die-Off Symptoms: Alka-Seltzer Gold, buffered vitamin C, activated charcoal, and Taheebo and grapefruit tea.

Headaches: Nystatin, vitamin E, vitamin C, vitamin B_3, coenzyme Q_{10}, evening primrose oil, and a calcium/magnesium supplement. One solution to migraine headaches brought on through exposure to chemicals or foods is to dissolve two Alka-Seltzer Gold tablets in water and drink the solution.

Leg/Muscle Cramps: Bioflavonoids, vitamin E, calcium/magnesium, vitamin B complex with extra niacin (vitamin B_3), and coenzyme Q_{10}.

Mental Fatigue: Diflucan, Ginkgo biloba, and coenzyme Q_{10}.

Physical Fatigue: Research shows that doses of about 2,500 to 5,000 micrograms of vitamin B_{12} administered by injection every two to three days helps CFS patients overcome physical fatigue. Magnesium and coenzyme Q_{10} are also helpful.

Premenstrual Syndrome: Calcium/magnesium, vitamin E, vitamin B_6, Ginkgo biloba, evening primrose oil, coenzyme Q_{10}, and zinc. Chasteberry, an herb often used to correct hormonal imbalances in women, is recommended for irregular or painful menstruation, PMS, and disorders connected to irregular hormone function.

Sugar Cravings: One item that can help cut down on sugar cravings for a short time is chromium picolinate, which is used by people with hypoglycemia. Patients should try 100 mg before each meal three times a day, and if this dose isn't enough, try 200 mg dose capsules. Since chromium picolinate is primarily grown on yeast, make sure you buy it in a yeast-free form.

Friendly Bacteria: Restoring Health with Probiotics

Probiotics are the beneficial bacteria inside us essential to good health. *Lactobacillus acidophilus* is perhaps the best known of the friendly bacteria and is commonly found in fresh yogurt. Studies done by Lance Peterson, M.D., formerly at the VA hospital in Minneapolis, found that the usual store-bought products have few "good guys" when the container has been left on the shelf for more than one week.

Often our digestive tract has been depleted of beneficial bacteria by antibiotics and other factors that help Candida get a position of power in our body. Without the protection of acidophilus and the other friendly bacteria, which actively defend their territory, Candida grows out of control. As Drs. Schmidt, Smith, and Sehnert write in *Beyond Antibiotics*:

> Another way that the normal intestinal bacteria protect against infection by invaders is simply by occupying space. They attach themselves to the wall of the intestine, leaving no available space to which parasites and other organisms can attach. If the good bacteria are eliminated, opportunists can move in and set up shop. The opportunists [such as Candida] compete with the other intestinal organisms for nutrients. Worse, they rob nutrients from the host. As they gain a stronger hold they make it easier for other members of their species to invade and get a foothold— they multiply.

In fact, the term *probiotics*, which means "for life," hints at the role of good bacteria in the body. Probiotic bacteria are both therapeutic and protective. Some help restore our health when it has been disrupted, and others help prevent disruption and illness. Some of the many functions of probiotics include:

- Helping reduce high cholesterol levels.
- Improving the efficiency of the digestive tract.
- Helping keep bowel functions at normal levels.
- Producing some of the B vitamins including biotin, pyridoxine (B_6), folic acid, and niacin (B_3).
- Excreting substances toxic to disease-causing bacteria.
- Protecting the body against toxic pollutants and radiation damage.

Besides these crucial functions, three kinds of probiotic bacteria help control the Candida organisms inside us and therefore promote recovery from CRC: *Lactobacillus acidophilus*, *Bifidobacterium bifidus*, and *Lactobacillus bulgaricus*. The more we learn about probiotic bacteria, the more they seem to irrevocably reflect either our good or bad health. In referring specifically to bifidobacterium, *Alternative Medicine: The Definitive Guide* by the Burton Goldberg Group writes, "There is strong evidence that the numbers and efficient working of these bacteria decline as a person ages and with any decline in our health status." Taking probiotic supplements both helps fight Candida organisms and helps restore the healthy ecology of your intestinal tract. Unfortunately, taking a few doses is not enough; they often have to be taken daily for several months. In *Back to Health,* Dr. Remington suggests acidophilus be taken for one month longer than the antifungal medication the patient is taking.

Correct usage of probiotics involves understanding how the different bacteria help the body and how to best keep them functioning properly. The main reasons *Lactobacillus acidophilus* and bifidobacterium are necessary are because they secrete antifungal substances that help destroy Candida organisms. Both are also essential to the normal health of the bowel.

Not surprisingly, the list of substances and conditions that decrease the effectiveness of probiotic bacteria is familiar: stress; a diet high in fatty meats, animal fats, cultured dairy products, and sugar; toxic pollutants; steroids; hormonal drugs such as birth control pills; and especially certain antibiotics. Probiotic bacteria are also less efficient and at decreased concentrations when large amounts of yeasts and bacteria are present in the body.

Lactobacillus acidophilus is the most common probiotic found in the small intestine and is also found in the mouth and vagina. One of the individual functions of acidophilus is to produce the enzyme lactase that helps the body digest the milk sugar found in dairy products. Some strains of acidophilus also produce their own form of chemical warfare in the form of natural antibiotics. Acidophilus creates lactic acid, which keeps the population of bad bacteria and yeasts under control.

One source of acidophilus is a milk found in some grocery stores called "sweet acidophilus" milk. Although yogurt is a natural source of acidophilus, most of the yogurts found in grocery stores are less a health food product and more a tasty sugar-filled treat. If you would like to eat yogurt a good idea is to buy a yogurt machine at a health food store or gourmet shop and make your own at home. The best choice, however, is acidophilus supplements that do not contain sugar and provide much higher doses of acidophilus than can be found in yogurt. When taking acidophilus supplements, be sure to start slowly with small doses to make sure the product agrees with you.

Bifidobacterium bifidus, also called bifidus, is the main resident of the large intestine in babies and children and is also found in the lower sections of the small intestine and in the vagina. Like acidophilus, bifidus prevents growth of disease-causing bacteria, some viruses, and yeasts (including Candida) partially by producing acetic acid. Bifidus also produces fatty acids such as caprylic acid, which is a naturally antifungal substance (discussed later in this chapter). Bifidus also helps to reduce liver stress by detoxifying ammonia in the colon. In addition, bifidus produces substances that help relieve constipation by directly stimulating intestinal function.

Bifidus is the main bacteria children need to have in their intestines and is passed from mother to child through breast milk. Children who are breast-fed have less intestinal infections because of the high amount of bifidus in their intestines.

Although *Lactobacillus bulgaricus*, the third useful probiotic, is transient, which means it doesn't permanently stay in the body, it is important because bulgaricus produces lactic acid, which helps provide an optimum environment for growth of acidophilus and bifidus.

Pay careful attention to the specific processes used in preparing probiotic supplements. Although only a few specific brands of probiotics meet the following requirements, when you consider that your recovery is at stake, it only makes sense to get the highest quality products available. When selecting quality freeze-dried probiotics look for this characteristic, which should be explained on the label: the filtration process. Do not buy probiotic supplements that have been prepared with a centrifuge, which swiftly spins the cultured liquid and damages the fragile chains of bacteria. Supplements that have been prepared using a slower process tend to be more expensive, but of higher quality. Some acidophilus supplements include DDS Acidophilus, Prime-Dophilus, Megadophilus, Maxidophilus, and Vital-Dophilus.

While the best form available for probiotics is the powdered form, often supplements are offered in capsules. The best kind of capsule is enteric-coated, which means it does not dissolve in the stomach, but rather in the intestines where the probiotics will do the most good. Probiotic supplements should also be stored in a dark glass, rather than a plastic container, and need to be refrigerated after opening. Probiotic supplements should not be taken near mealtimes because when food is present in the stomach, the levels of acidity increase, thereby decreasing the supplement's potency.

Natural Remedies for Treating CRC

Natural remedies are important both for patients who would like to avoid prescription medications if possible and as part of a complete approach for patients already taking prescription medications. Following one part of the recovery program is never enough. Complete recovery is impossible without at least two things: strict adherence to the Candida control diet and antifungal medications of some kind. The best approach is one that includes some of all of the treatments available, no matter how difficult or inconvenient they may be.

Just as the symptoms of CRC vary from person to person, so do the effectiveness and suitability of the remedies listed in this section. Many patients find Taheebo tea helpful, others don't. Some are helped by caprylic acid, while others don't notice a change in their health.

Even though these remedies, medications, or food substances are available without a prescription and easily found in your local pharmacy or health food store, do not underestimate their potency or potential for harm. As with all medications, side effects are as possible as beneficial effects, so be sure to follow the instructions on the label. It is also a good idea to speak to your physician before adding another medication, food substance, or nutritional supplement to your treatment regimen.

Except in some specific instances, dosage information for the treatments described in this chapter has not been included. There are two reasons for this: the potency and size of the supplements vary from brand to brand; and your physician should be your primary guide for medication because he has the latest available information and is familiar with your individual case.

Nonprescription Antifungals

A wide variety of effective and natural nonprescription antifungal medicines that specifically kill Candida are available and include caprylic acid, garlic, citrus seed extract, Taheebo tea, Mathake tea, and Tanalbit.

As previously mentioned, it is a good idea to supplement your treatment regimen with nonprescription antifungal medications regardless of whether or not you are taking prescription medications. As with prescription antifungal medications, die-off symptoms are also possible with the use of nonprescription antifungal remedies. To lessen die-off reactions, begin by taking small doses and work up to larger amounts.

If you have problems tolerating either the prescription medications or the die-off side effects from prescription medicines, you may want to discontinue medication for a short time and try the natural antifungals listed in this chapter. After several weeks or months when large amounts of Candida have been destroyed, speak to your physician about the possibility of starting a regimen of prescription antifungal drugs.

The following is a list of useful nonprescription antifungal treatments.

Caprylic Acid: One extremely safe and effective antifungal substance commonly used to treat overgrowth is caprylic acid. If you have irritable bowel syndrome (IBS) don't take caprylic acid without first speaking with your doctor.

Some physicians who prefer to avoid use of prescription antifungal medicines unless they are absolutely necessary first start their patients on caprylic acid supplements and then move to prescription medicines if no improvement is made. No side effects other than occasional digestive problems have been reported, although, as with any antifungal medication or treatment regimen, die-off symptoms are normal.

Caprylic acid is a naturally occurring short-chain saturated fatty acid. Although it is a potent antifungal, the exact mechanism by which it impairs or kills fungal cells is unknown. The usual dose is one to two capsules with every meal, but if you are just beginning to take caprylic acid, start at a lower dose and speak with your physician. Common brand names for caprylic acid supplements include Mycopryl 400 or 680 and Kaprycidin A.

For maximum effect be sure to take time-release or enteric-coated capsules to slow down the release of caprylic acid into the intestinal tract. Some examples of time-release or enteric-coated caprylic acid supplements are Caprinex, Candistat, Caprystatin, and Capricin. Whether or not you should take caprylic acid supplements on a full or empty stomach varies from supplement to supplement, so be sure to read the label directions. As with any product described in this book, consult your physician if you are pregnant or nursing.

Garlic: Another powerful anti-Candida substance is garlic, which, because of its antifungal, antiviral, and antibacterial properties, has been used to treat illnesses around the world for thousands of years. From ancient to modern times, garlic has been a favored choice among physicians who prefer natural treatments. Both Virgil and Hippocrates mention garlic as treatments for snakebite and pneumonia, and enough scientific interest has created the need for entire conferences on the efficacy of garlic, such as the 1990 World Congress on Garlic, attended by more than fifty scientists from fifteen countries. Since 1960, more than one thousand research papers on garlic's curative effects against cancer, infectious diseases, and heart disease have been published in medical journals. Studies have also shown one-half to one clove of garlic per day reduces blood cholesterol levels by 9 percent. A study on the effects of garlic against Candida showed garlic helped clear Candida cells from the blood and reduced the amount of Candida growth in the kidney.

The main curative component in garlic appears to be allicin, which has been proven effective against a large list of microbes including *E. coli, Salmonella, Candida albicans*, and others. Although allicin seems to be the active ingredient, garlic supplements that lack allicin are still effective, indicating that more than one ingredient is important. Studies have, in fact, revealed that garlic is a more effective remedy for sore throats than penicillin, and that one milligram of allicin is equal to fifteen standard units of penicillin.

Garlic cloves do not have to be eaten whole or raw; in fact, raw garlic is more likely to cause allergic reactions than cooked garlic. Chopping, steaming, or cooking garlic, as well as the odor or lack of odor, such as in deodorized garlic capsules, does not decrease the potency or effects of garlic. When buying fresh garlic, examine the head or bulb to make sure it is firm and compact. If there are sprouts, the garlic is too old. It is also important to store fresh garlic in a cool, airy, dry place, not in the refrigerater and not in a plastic bag or other airtight container. Under ideal circumstances garlic will stay fresh for up to six months. Studies show that to be effective garlic should be taken every day.

Another way to benefit from the healing properties of garlic is to extract your own garlic oil in the same fashion as the manufacturers of garlic supplements, but on a smaller scale. In *The Candida Albicans*

Yeast-Free Cookbook Pat Connolly tells readers how to do it: add one cup of vodka or gin to one-half pound peeled garlic cloves and blend the ingredients in a blender. Add a second cup of liquor and continue to blend until the mixture has the consistency of mush. After pouring the mush into a quart jar, rinse the blender with one-third cup of liquor and add this to the mixture in the jar. Be sure to tightly cap the jar and to shake it daily, just long enough to make sure the alcohol and mush mix. After shaking the mixture for ten days, about an inch of garlic oil should rise to the top. Carefully skim it off. Just remove the oil; do not extract any of the original garlic mash. Every time you remove oil, add a little more liquor. When no more oil appears, discard the mash and start over again.

Unfortunately, none of the supplements available seems to contain as much garlic as the fresh version. When selecting garlic supplements you may want to avoid garlic oils because they do not seem to contain very much actual garlic. Steam-distilled garlic oil capsules contain 1 percent garlic compounds and 99 percent vegetable oil; garlic oil macerate capsules also contain exceedingly small amounts of garlic extract. Garlic powder pills and aged garlic tablets and liquid seem to be the best alternatives besides fresh garlic. Although many brands are available and are no doubt effective to certain extents, one brand in particular, Kyolic, an aged and deodorized garlic extract, seems to be a popular choice among physicians, scientists, and patients, even though it doesn't contain allicin. One effective garlic supplement that retains the allicin is Garlicin by Nature's Way Products.

Citrus Seed Extract: Widely used because of its antimicrobial activities to prevent spoilage in food, citrus seed extract is derived from grapefruit seeds, and has the potential to be a very powerful medication for a variety of illnesses. Besides effectively killing bacteria, citrus seed extract is also a formidable broad-spectrum antifungal that is extremely effective against Candida. In fact, citrus seed extract is currently used to treat Candida infections of the intestines as well as other intestinal problems. In *The Yeast Connection and the Woman,* Dr. Crook reports that citrus seed extract is as effective an antifungal as nystatin and caprylic acid.

Citrus seed extract has been used outside the U.S. to treat a variety of illnesses for many years. It is also being tested by the Pasteur Institute in France as a possible agent against the HIV virus responsible for AIDS. Only recently has citrus seed extract been used in the United States for medicinal purposes. Citrus seed extract is available in capsules and liquid. Some citrus seed extract brand names that you should be able to find in your health food store are Citricidal and ParaMicrocidin.

Taheebo Tea: Another antifungal substance and healing aid is Taheebo tea, also called La Pacho or Pau d'arco tea. The tea comes from the inner bark of two South American trees (the Lapacho Colorado and the Lapacho Marado) that have been used medicinally by the native populations in the Andes for hundreds of years. The bark of these trees has long been used to treat infections, intestinal complaints, and ailments such as cystitis and prostatitis. This type of bark is reported to be analgesic, an antiviral, a diuretic, and a fungicide.

According to a 1983 article in *The Human Ecologist* written by Gail Fraser Nielsen, "The benefits from drinking the tea appear to be subtle. Patients report suddenly being aware that they're less sensitive to molds, chemicals, and/or foods. They state that although they are experiencing localized symptoms, their general feeling of physical and mental well-being has been enhanced."

Although Taheebo tea is perhaps the best known tea used by CRC patients, other teas are available, such as Mathake tea, an inexpensive herbal product that can be helpful when used as part of a treatment regimen that includes the diet and prescription and nonprescription medications. Jack Parker, a pharmacist who owns and runs a health food store in upstate New York, recommends and sells a daily tea for Candida made of Pau d'arco, echinacea, lemon grass, peppermint, hibiscus flowers, rose hips, cinnamon, licorice root, and stevia.

Tanalbit: Tanalbit, which comes in capsule form, contains tannic acid, a natural substance found in nature. When tannic acid is combined with zinc, an antifungal substance called zinc-salicylo-tannate, which is effective in treating Candida, is formed. Tanalbit has been described as an internal intestinal antiseptic. Besides fighting intestinal overgrowth of Candida, it also relieves gastrointestinal problems, such as acute and chronic diarrhea, constipation, spastic colon, and colitis.

According to Luc De Schepper, M.D., Ph.D., author of *Candida*, Tanalbit "is not a first-line drug such as the Caprycillic [sic.] acid preparations, but it is certainly a valid alternative for people who cannot handle the die-off symptoms." It is also recommended for patients who do not benefit from caprylic acid supplements. There are no known side effects.

Tanalbit is usually taken with meals for several months. It is manufactured by the Scientific Consulting Service, a company that supplies nutritional products ([800]-333-7414).

Substances that Boost the Immune System
Vitamin and nutrient supplements are essential for recovery from Candida overgrowth because Candida depletes the body of essential

nutrients and impairs the immune system. Although many vitamins and minerals can boost the immune system, specific information on only a few are presented.

In a perfect world we would all get the vitamins and minerals we need from the foods we eat every day. Since we live in a far from perfect world, vitamin/mineral supplements are an extremely important part of a full recovery from CRC. But even eating a balanced and highly nutritious diet wouldn't give each of us the amount of vitamins our bodies need. In fact, increasing vitamin intake through diet alone is almost impossible. For example, you would have to eat the following to reach recommended daily allowances:

- Fifteen oranges every day to get 1,000 mg of vitamin C.

- Twenty-four cups of almonds to get enough vitamin E.

- Five cups of carrots and six cups of butternut squash to get enough beta carotene.

Since dietary sources are not enough, obtaining vitamins and minerals through supplements is a reasonable alternative. When taking supplements be sure to take them after eating, not on an empty stomach. And when shopping for your supplements, be careful to choose supplements that are sugar-, yeast-, and color-free.

Vitamins that help rebuild a weakened immune system include the following:

- Vitamin A, which increases immune response and helps the body build resistance to infection.

- The individual B vitamins, which increase antibody response. One in particular is vitamin B_6, the antistress vitamin, which is necessary for normal function of the GI tract and which helps in treatment of anxiety and depression.

- Vitamins C and E, which are essential to normal immune system function.

- Beta carotene, which also helps the immune system fight infection.

Other crucial nutrients that help a body exhausted by CRC include antioxidant immune boosters, such as calcium, selenium, and zinc, and adrenal stimulants, such as glandular adrenal (an extract), chromium, and magnesium. To help restore your immune system so it can respond to the Candida overgrowth, take the following daily doses of necessary supplements:

8 to 10 grams of vitamin C

250 mg of vitamin B_5 (pantothenic acid)

500 to 1,000 mg of taurine

25 to 50 mg of zinc chelate

250 mg of goldenseal root extract twice a day. Make sure you buy goldenseal root extract that contains no less than 5 percent hydrastine.

The suggested dosages of vitamins and minerals for adults vary from health professional to health professional. In *The Yeast Connection and the Woman*, Dr. Crook recommends these vitamin/mineral supplements for patients with Candida-related problems:

5,000 to 10,000 IU of vitamin A	100 mg of inositol
100 to 200 micrograms of selenium	50 mg of PABA
200 to 800 micrograms of folic acid	15 to 30 mg of zinc
100 micrograms of vitamin B_{12}	1 to 2 mg of copper
300 micrograms of biotin	20 mg of manganese
100 micrograms of choline (bitartrate)	100 mg of citrus bioflavonoids
100 to 400 IU of vitamin D	200 micrograms of chromium
400 to 600 IU of vitamin E	500 mg of calcium
100 micrograms of molybdenum	1 mg of boron
25 micrograms of vanadium	500 mg of magnesium
25 to 100 mg of vitamin B_1	100 to 500 mg pantothenic acid
25 to 50 mg of vitamin B_{21}	100 to 150 mg of niacinamide
25 to 100 mg of vitamin B_6	

Coenzyme Q_{10} (CoQ_{10}): Coenzyme Q_{10}, also known as ubiquinone, is a nutrient that strengthens and plays a crucial role in the function of the immune system and aids circulation and metabolic function. It is an antioxidant that is similar to vitamin E, but suspected to be more powerful.

Among its other many benefits, CoQ_{10} is frequently used to treat patients with congestive heart failure and other types of heart disease. It has an extremely bright future, including a possible help for AIDS and cancer. According to *Prescription for Nutritional Healing* by James F. Balch, M.D., and Phyllis A. Balch, C.N.C., "The use of Coenzyme Q_{10} is a major step forward in the prevention and control of cancer." Coenzyme Q_{10} is often recommended by physicians to patients with chronic infections.

Echinacea: Extract from the roots and leaves of the echinacea plant is one of the most popular herbs used to boost the immune system and combat colds and flus. According to Drs. Schmidt, Smith, and Sehnert, authors of *Beyond Antibiotics*, "This is one of the most widely used and heavily studied immune-boosting herbs in the world." In addition to its powerful immune-system stimulants, echinacea also has antiviral, antibiotic, and anti-inflammatory properties and has been used effectively to treat Candida infections. In fact, according to Drs. Schmidt, Smith, and Sehnert, "It [echinacea] was also shown to be a 30 percent more potent T-cell stimulator than the most potent T-cell stimulator known at this time."

Essential Fatty Acids (EFAs): Not all dietary fats are bad. Some, such as essential fatty acids, provide necessary nutrients the body cannot manufacture on its own and therefore must be added through a complete diet. EFAs play an important role in the body by doing the following:

- Strengthening the immune system.
- Being an integral part of the cell wall of every cell in the body.
- Helping with various biochemical processes.
- Providing the raw elements the body needs to make prosta-glandins, which are the message carriers manufactured by all cells throughout the body.

EFAs can be obtained from two different sources: plants and their seeds and cold-water fish. Unprocessed vegetable oils that contain EFAs are linseed, safflower, sesame (not the Oriental variety), corn, primrose, and sunflower oils. Other rich sources are flaxseeds, walnuts, canola oil, and fish such as salmon, sardines, tuna, mackerel, menhaden, and herring. Although diabetics cannot take fish-oil supplements, they can eat fish.

EFAs, which are polyunsaturated, can be divided into two different types of essential fatty acids: Omega 3, also called linolenic acid, and Omega 6, also known as linoleic acid. Omega 3 oils are used to help relieve symptoms of PMS and to treat all major degenerative diseases, including arthritis, heart disease, cancer, and multiple sclerosis. Both are extremely beneficial to the body.

Since fish found in cold, deep water have a higher fat content (as insulation against the cold), they contain more Omega 3 fatty acids. For example, four ounces of salmon, a cold-water fish, can contain thirty-six hundred milligrams, while four ounces of cod, a low-fat fish, can contain only three hundred milligrams of Omega 3 fatty acids.

Both types of EFAs can be purchased in capsule form, but be sure to check the expiration date because they can become rancid. Flaxseeds and flax oil contain the highest concentration of Omega 3 fatty acids of any other known source, but can also become rancid and should therefore be stored in dark glass bottles and refrigerated. Flaxseed has a nutty taste and can be mixed with a variety of liquids including water and fruit or vegetable juices. Flaxseed can also be added to soups, salads, cereals, and yogurt. Evening primrose oil and black currant seed oil are excellent sources of Omega 6 fatty acids. The recommended dosage of Omega 6 fatty acids for someone with CRC would be about six to eight capsules of evening primrose oil per day.

Improving Digestion Helps Lessen Symptoms and Ultimately CRC

Everything begins with digestion. Eating nutritious foods won't help if the nutrients processed from the food aren't distributed throughout the body. "You can't get the nutrients you need if your digestion isn't working properly," said Pauline, a CRC patient who emphasizes the need for digestive enzymes (in chapter 16). Some of the common signs of food malabsorption are also frequent CRC symptoms, such as abdominal pain, diarrhea, fatigue, impotence, and irritable bowels. Common clinical problems that can be related to malabsorption and are associated with CRC are acne, constipation, diarrhea, eczema, impaired immunity, food allergies, mineral deficiencies, and leaky gut syndrome. Taking antacids to alleviate gastric symptoms can be counterproductive since they reduce the hydrochloric acid necessary for digestion.

One of the main functions of the GI tract is to break down molecules and absorb nutrients. A GI tract impaired by Candida overgrowth cannot fully digest foods, which is why digestive enzymes help. Enzymes are responsible for every chemical reaction in the body, and without enzymes the raw materials we ingest such as proteins, carbohydrates, and fats would be useless because they cannot be split into useable parts.

Candida overgrowth hinders the effectiveness of the GI tract, negatively affecting the digestive process. Because the body is overtaxed by Candida overgrowth it can't produce its own enzymes. Digestive enzyme supplements help both by aiding digestion and by taking stress off the organs of the body that produce enzymes. When digestion is improved, unpleasant symptoms decrease and the immune system is able to function better. In fact, when digestive problems are straightened out and absorption of essential nutrients is achieved through use of enzymes, patients with many chronic conditions report improvement.

There are two types of enzymes—plant-derived and pancreatic—and they can be used independently or together. Plant enzymes improve digestion by predigesting the food. This eases the workload of the body, which in turn strengthens the digestive system. Pancreatic enzymes are often derived from animal enzymes and aid the digestion of food once it has reached the intestinal tract and lower stomach. Pancreatic enzymes help both the digestive and immune systems and can alleviate multiple food allergies.

It is important to note that enzyme therapy will not help unless combined with proper eating habits and the diet. Also, be sure you are getting enough vitamin B_{12} (cyanocobalamin) because the body needs it to properly digest and absorb foods. In order to be most effective, digestive enzymes should be taken with meals, not after a meal is finished.

Hydrochloric acid is also crucial to digestion and can be taken in capsule form to increase deficient hydrochloric acid in the stomach. Be sure you take the capsule form and not the liquid form because the liquid form can damage your teeth. Check with your doctor before taking hydrochloric acid supplements if you are taking azole drugs

Deficiencies of hydrochloric acid are often found in CRC patients and are probably at least partially responsible for the digestive problems and gastrointestinal symptoms frequently reported by CRC patients. Not only does a lack of hydrochloric acid in the stomach hinder digestion, it also permits Candida overgrowth. In addition, nutrient deficiencies, aging, and food allergies can decrease the amount of hydrochloric acid in the stomach. Two vitamins that help the body produce hydrochloric acid are vitamin B_1 (thiamine) and vitamin B_6 (pyridoxine).

Colon Health: An Important Step toward Recovery

One extremely effective way to lessen the symptoms of die-off and to aid in your recovery in general is to keep your colon as free of toxins (especially Candida toxins) as possible. One way to do this is by eating a high-fiber diet. Another is to undergo a procedure called colonic hydrotherapy or colonic irrigation. Before starting this or any therapy, be sure to ask your physician which treatments will best help your unique situation.

A High-Fiber Diet Is Essential for Optimum Colon Health

A high-fiber diet helps promote regular bowel movements, which means toxins are efficiently eliminated from the body. A high-fiber diet contains roughage, which is grain fibers and other insoluble substances the colon finds easier to move forward than other substances. As a result there is a shorter transit time between the consumption and elimination of food, and the patient has more regular bowel movements.

Because fiber can't be digested by the body, it helps move waste substances through the intestines. Grain fibers, such as rice bran or wheat, also absorb water. Crude fibers such as mucilages, gums, and pectins (which are found in many fruits) both soften the bowel movement and may even help lengthen nutrient transport time in the GI tract.

Studies have found that the benefits of a high-fiber diet are numerous and include inhibiting excessive growth of bacteria in the colon. Also, because fiber stretches out the colon, it allows fewer carcinogens to attach to the walls of the intestines. Fiber may also inhibit the absorption of cholesterol. Foods high in fiber include oat bran, rice bran, brown rice, fruits, vegetables, and nuts.

In a 1991 interview published in *Health Counselor*, Terry Lemerond, president and founder of Enzymatic Therapy in Wisconsin, describes fiber as a broom that sweeps material through the system. In commenting on how to detoxify the body naturally, he recommends that patients follow a diet that doesn't disrupt the body. Lemerond suggests lightly steamed and nonstarchy vegetables, salads, fresh fruits, and food high in high-quality protein, such as cold-water fish (which also provide essential fatty acids) and chicken.

Fiber supplements are available, and Lemerond recommends buying those with water-soluble fibers such as oat bran and psyllium. Other important water-soluble fibers include guar gum, karaya gum, dandelion root powder, apple pectin, fennel seed powder, ginger root powder, fenugreek, and sarsaparilla root powder. Water-soluble fibers are essential because they can bind with poisons, fats, and heavy metals and remove them from the system.

When trying to eliminate toxins from the body, it is also important to drink plenty of water. Water removes toxins while cleansing the interior of the body. At least two quarts of purified water per day is highly recommended. Two other enjoyable ways to rid the body of toxins are through exercise and sauna baths. Exercise helps remove toxins by speeding oxygen to the cells. About twenty minutes of vigorous walking a day is usually sufficient. Saunas are beneficial because they induce sweating, which is a natural way the body excretes toxins.

Colonic Hydrotherapy: An Excellent Way to Remove Candida Toxins

Colonic hydrotherapy, often called colonic irrigation, is another extremely efficient way to remove Candida toxins from the body. Colonic hydrotherapy involves introducing water into the colon and allowing the natural peristaltic muscle to remove fecal matter. This procedure is repeated several times over a period of forty-five minutes to an hour and is done with sterilized and FDA-approved equipment. Often two to three visits a week are needed to completely cleanse and tone the colon.

Colonic hydrotherapy is available throughout the United States and Canada as well as in other countries. It is legal in every state in this country. According to the International Association for Colon Therapy (which certifies colon hydrotherapists) based in Redding, California, states with high percentages of colon hydrotherapists are Texas, Michigan, New York, Florida, Illinois, California, Arizona, Nevada, Washington, and New Mexico.

Colonic hydrotherapy is especially useful in the early stages of CRC treatment and during the die-off period due to the excessive amounts of toxins released by the Candida organisms when they die in large quantities. This procedure is also highly recommended for patients who have problems with constipation. Not all people should undergo colonic hydrotherapy. Patients in a very weakened state should not attempt colonic hydrotherapy without medical supervision. Patients with specific medical conditions such as ulcerative colitis, Crohn's disease (in the acute inflammatory state), tumors of the large intestine or rectum, diverticulitis, and severe hemorrhoids should also not attempt colonic hydrotherapy.

The colon is a segment of the large intestine, or bowel, and varies in length from about 1.5 to 1.8 meters long. Colonic hydrotherapy is not and should not be considered an enema. An enema reaches only the sigmoid colon, which is the lower eight to twelve inches of the bowel. Colonic hydrotherapy allows the water to travel the entire length of the large bowel.

Patients who undergo colonic hydrotherapy occasionally have some side effects, including brief feelings of nausea and diarrhea. According to *Alternative Medicine: The Definitive Guide*, it is a good idea to eat and drink lightly and, especially if you are constipated, to give yourself an enema before undergoing colonic hydrotherapy. "An enema beforehand will empty the rectum and increase the efficiency of the colon therapy. After colon therapy, gentle, nourishing foods should be taken, such as vegetable soups and broths and fruits and vegetable juices."

Choosing a Reputable Colonic Hydrotherapist

Although colonic hydrotherapy is a perfectly legal procedure in the United States, colon hydrotherapists do not have to be certified except in Florida, which is the only state that requires practitioners to be licensed under the board of massage and then certified in colon hydrotherapy. Because of this, and because fecal matter can transmit diseases, it is extremely important to be careful when selecting a colon therapist.

There have been very few problems in the past regarding the proper sanitation of equipment, and according to a 1994 article in the *Washington Post*, colon therapists report that complications are extremely rare today. The reasons for this include improved sterilization procedures and disposable tubes and other equipment. The same article also reported that the FDA has never received any complaints regarding enema devices. In fact, the International Association for Colon Therapy reported that in its six years in business, it has received only three complaints regarding certified colon hydrotherapists and none of these complaints concerned improper sanitation.

The International Association for Colon Therapy is an association that provides services such as education, training, and certification for colon therapists. The association also provides assistance for patients. These services include referrals to certified colon therapists in their area and a list of questions patients should ask a colon therapist when investigating the therapist and his or her establishment. Dollie Popoff, a staff secretary for the association, said that when inspecting a colon therapist and his or her establishment, patients should primarily look for a sterile and clean environment. The organization or establishment itself should be clean and orderly, and the table the procedure is performed on should be immaculate. You should also be given your own gown.

The most important cleanliness factor, however, is the condition of the colonic hydrotherapy equipment. It is essential that the disposable waste hoses be changed for every patient. Popoff said patients should actually see the disposable hose taken out of a plastic bag in front of them. A hose that has been previously used, even if it has been cleaned by the practitioner or an assistant, is completely and thoroughly unacceptable. If the colon hydrotherapist uses stainless steel speculums, it is important to note the sanitation procedure used by the therapist. A germicide and auto-clave system should be used correctly. In addition, Popoff stressed that patients should investigate to make sure their colon therapist is certified by either a state school or by a reputable organization.

For a referral to a certified colon therapist, call the International Association for Colon Therapy at (916) 222-1498, or write them at 2051 Hilltop Dr., Suite A-11, Redding, CA 96002. The American Association of Naturopathic Physicians can also refer you to a qualified colon hydrotherapist. Their phone number is (206) 323-7610, and their address is 2366 Eastlake Ave., Suite 322, Seattle, Wa, 98102.

The advice in this chapter has helped many patients not only control their health on a daily basis, but also boost their immune systems to the point where it can help them overcome their health problems. The remedies listed in this chapter are as crucial to your recovery as the prescription antifungal medications and the Candida control diet.

—12—

What to Do if You Aren't Getting Better

Pain, messenger of harm
Nature's poignant alarm
Often man's wily friend
To signal means to mend.
—David Seegal in *The Pharos of Alpha Omega Alpha*

Just as CRC generally develops over a period of many months or years, treatment can also take time and be difficult. Some patients who take antifungal medications and follow the diet are able to get their CRC under control within a brief period of time, although they cannot return to a lifestyle that includes antibiotics, birth control pills, or large amounts of sugar. Other patients are not as successful and may need months or years to regain their health.

While many of the books and articles on CRC are full of patient success stories, not all patients recover from CRC. In *The Yeast Connection*, Dr. Crook writes that about 90 percent of the hundreds of patients he has treated with Candida-related illnesses have improved. Overall, many patients make rapid improvements in the first few months after beginning treatment, and then their rate of improvement slows down. Other patients do not improve beyond a certain point. As Dr. Remington explains, "Many people are 50 to 75 percent improved after three months, but require another year or more to improve all the way. Some people aren't 100 percent better even after an entire year."

When discussing the difficulties sometimes associated with overcoming Candida-related illnesses Dr. Crook emphasizes the importance of patience and time. As Dr. Crook writes, "strengthening the

151

immune system and regaining health may occasionally be quick and easy. *More often, it takes time, patience, persistence and careful management of the multiple factors contributing to the illness."*

Possible Explanations for Slow Progress

Although there are an endless number of possible reasons for a patient's lack of improvement or inability to completely recover from CRC, several explanations are more likely than others. These possible reasons are provided as guidelines only. Remember, your physician is your best source for answers since he is familiar with your individual health problems, your treatments, and the latest medical information.

In addition to the external factors needed to recover from any illness—the medications, supplements, or other remedies involved—recovery from any illness depends on you helping your body help itself. All medicines, exercises, and nutritious foods have one purpose and goal: to strengthen the body to the point where it can take care of the infection or problem by itself. If you aren't recovering, something is weakening your immune system so that it cannot do its job.

If you aren't improving, your first step should be to have a lengthy and thorough discussion with your physician. Describe the symptoms you still have, the treatments you have found to be helpful or unhelpful, and what you consider to be an ideal state of health. Be clear about what you expect and need from your physician so there will be less chance of a misunderstanding and so you and your physician can successfully work together to resolve your health problems. You may also want to seek a second opinion from another doctor.

After considering your situation, your physician might decide additional health problems are unlikely and suggest the best idea is to simply alter your CRC treatment. Changing your treatment might include increasing the doses of your medications, trying new medications, adding more supplements to your treatment regimen, or further restricting your diet. As mentioned in chapter 8, one common reason patients relapse or fail to fully recover is because they try to control their CRC through diet alone. Antifungal medications greatly aid recovery by helping clear Candida out of the tissues of the body.

Another possibility is you might have Chronic Fatigue Syndrome (CFS), which causes symptoms similar to CRC. Speak to your physician about being tested for CFS. When you visit your physician you will probably need a complete physical examination as well.

If your health has greatly improved, but you occasionally have symptoms, this isn't always a cause for alarm. Two possible explanations could be hidden or delayed food allergies. Both food sensitivities and delayed food allergies can cause a wide variety of symptoms, such as headaches, abdominal pain, depression, anxiety, sinus pain, digestive disorders, and many others. Sensitivities to common foods, sometimes called hidden or delayed food allergies, could be causing discomfort. Some common foods known to cause sensitivities are chocolate, citrus fruits, milk, wheat, corn, food colorings, and other food additives. Delayed food allergies tend to appear several hours or days after the food is eaten. If you suspect that food allergies might be your problem, try excluding foods you suspect you might be allergic to, eliminating all foods you habitually crave, and rotating your diet.

If your symptoms last for one to two weeks a month they could actually be intense premenstrual syndrome symptoms. Another possibility is that even though you are following all the treatments for CRC, stress in your life could be keeping you from completely recovering. Stress is often connected with the onset of illness and the body's inability to recover.

There could be any number of reasons why you still haven't recovered. In addition to those discussed above, the physicians who treat this condition have repeatedly found four common hindrances to recovery, which follow:

- Chronic exposure to mold in your home or workplace.
- Chronic exposure to chemicals in your home or workplace.
- The possibility that you might have parasites.
- Toxins released into your body from mercury-silver amalgam dental fillings.

Mold: A Common Problem in the Home
Most of us have had limited experiences with mold and think of it as dark goo on the bathroom tile or greenish stuff on last month's leftovers in the refrigerator. Unfortunately for all of us, these obvious forms of mold are not the only examples of mold in the home. Technically, mold is any type of fungus growth that usually causes destruction of organic matter. Most mold is microscopic and therefore difficult to detect. In general, any place that is damp or dark is an ideal place for mold growth. Mold grows best in places where air circulation is poor. The best way to combat mold is to prevent it from growing. This is done by using simple common-sense methods to improve the air quality in your home and by removing materials that can harbor mold or facilitate mold growth.

Common places mold can be found in the home are bathrooms, basements, kitchens, attics, air vents and ducts, humidifiers, old books and magazines, and poorly ventilated closets or rooms. If you own a clothes dryer, be sure to vent it to the outside of the house. Other sources include old furnishings and home decorations, such as beds and bedding, carpets, any leather objects, furniture, and wallpaper. Mold can also be found on fruits and vegetables, in the soil, and on plants both in the house and outside and on dried flowers. Mold is also present in the air in the form of spores. Spores make it possible for mold to survive under less-than-perfect living conditions and are the way in which mold reproduces. As Drs. Schmidt, Smith, and Sehnert note in *Beyond Antibiotics*, "Mold is an insidious culprit that can permeate the home and be a constant source of immune system stress." Common allergic symptoms that may indicate the presence of mold in your home are severe allergic reactions and impaired breathing.

If you are having trouble recovering from CRC, thoroughly investigate the possibility that a mold problem at your house or workplace is delaying your recovery. Many CRC patients have found that their CRC symptoms greatly improve after leaving moldy houses and/or relocating to drier climates.

Exposure to mold increases and intensifies CRC symptoms and depresses the immune system. Plus, because their immune systems are already weakened, CRC patients are more sensitive to mold than healthy people are. As Dr. Lorenzani explains in *Candida: A Twentieth Century Disease*, "[A negative reaction to mold] can mean that your immune system, which in a healthy state could deal with common household fungi, is depressed by fungi growing within your body. Because of that depression of your immune system, you are now reacting to common household fungi and molds which normally would not bother you."

Patients with allergies often find that their allergies are aggravated by the presence of mold. In a 1982 article in the *Annals of Allergy*, Fred Terracina, Ph.D., and Sherry A. Rogers, M.D., cite the statistic that 86 percent of patients with inhalant allergies also had mold allergies. "Airborne fungi are frequently associated with allergic manifestations," they add.

Mold and mildew in our homes may be more prevalent than previously realized. A 1991 article in the *American Journal of Public Health* reported findings by Canadian researchers that show that out of fifteen thousand homes studied, a full 32.4 percent had mold, 21.4 percent had flooding, and 14.1 percent had moisture from other sources. Although the climates in the United States and Canada are different, these statistics are worth noting. Blair, one woman with CRC (featured in chapter 16), said that during her childhood she lived in a house that had a severe mildew problem. "It was on all the walls and we just kept painting over it," she said. "We didn't know any better." Many CRC patients report their symptoms become worse during damp or rainy weather. One reason for this is mold spores multiply more rapidly in damp weather.

The best way to get rid of mold in your home is to make the environment as unfavorable to mold growth as possible by keeping damp places dry and dark areas well-lit. One way to keep dampness under control is to frequently air out rooms and to use a dehumidifier, a machine that removes moisture from the air. Since closets often develop mold, leave a light on in your closets at all times or install a louvered door. There are many things you can do in the kitchen to help prevent mold from growing: always cover steaming pots, don't let faucets run needlessly, and if you have a fan above your stove turn it on when cooking. In general, it's best not to keep house plants, and if you have an aquarium, keep it covered. A boric solution can be used to topically treat moldy areas around the house. Be sure to throw away any items that you suspect harbor mold.

Chemicals in Your Home or Workplace

Just as chemicals can contribute to the onset of CRC, chronic exposure to chemicals in your environment can keep you from fully recovering. A detailed explanation of chemicals and how they can damage the body can be found in chapter 5. We all have individual toxic loads, which describes the level of toxic substances our bodies can handle without harm. If our exposure to chemicals exceeds these limits, we become ill. As we all know, chemicals are all around us: in our food, clothing, homes, cars, personal-care products, and in every aspect of our lives. Constant contact with chemicals further weakens the immune systems of patients who are already very sensitive to their surrounding and increases or prolongs symptoms.

Just as with exposure to mold, when some patients decrease their exposure to chemicals, their symptoms decrease and their health improves. The presence of substances that continually aggravate your body and your health affects your immune system negatively. Often the removal of these aggravating factors is exactly what your body needs to begin correcting the imbalances in it. Changing your environment may seem like a big price to pay, especially if you are accustomed to living with the symptoms of your CRC, but when you realize just how precious health is and exactly what is at stake, you will be able to make the necessary, and sometimes difficult, changes in your life.

Parasites: A Complication for Some CRC Patients

The presence of parasites in a patient can make CRC difficult to treat. An article in the *Journal of Alternative and Complementary Medicine* states that it is believed Candida infections can become resistant to treatment because of parasites, such as amoebas, nematodes, *Giardia lamblia*, and cestodes.

There are many tests for parasites, including blood, urine, and stool tests. One problem with testing for parasites is the failure of some labs to detect parasites in the samples sent to them. One way to increase your chances of getting a correct diagnosis is to make sure your doctor, hospital, or diagnostic laboratory follows the guidelines set by the *Manual of Clinical Microbiology* and the Centers for Disease Control for the testing of intestinal parasites. A new method of testing for parasites, called immunofluorescent staining, shows remarkable promise by making parasites easier to see in the lab specimens. One lab that uses such staining is Great Smokies Diagnostic Laboratory in North Carolina.

How could you have developed a parasitic infection? Common sources of parasites include pets, the water we drink, and the food we eat. Our pets, especially cats and dogs, may carry a variety of worms or other parasitic organisms. To avoid picking up a parasite from your pets, wash your hands frequently and speak to your veterinarian about prophylactic parasitic treatments.

Surprisingly enough, parasites can be found in drinking water if the cysts (or eggs) haven't been properly filtered out. Water from rivers, lakes, and streams may also be contaminated with single-celled parasitic organisms. Although you may not intentionally drink water from these sources, if you participate in outdoor water sports, such as water skiing, swimming, canoeing, or any other similar sports, you may accidentally swallow infected water.

Perhaps the most common source of parasites is from contaminated food, specifically raw meat. When raw, the following foods may contain a variety of parasites: fish, beef, pork, lamb, and horse meat. Raw oysters, mussels, and clams, especially those from the east coast of the United States, also can be contaminated with a wide variety of parasites. Raw chicken can carry bacteria and viruses and sometimes parasites. Vegetables especially can also harbor parasites.

The best way to avoid parasites is to thoroughly cook your food and never eat anything raw, especially fish because it usually contains worms. Be sure to wash your hands after handling raw meat, and do not put your hands near your mouth. Avoid contaminating the surfaces of your kitchen, and thoroughly wash the utensils you use to cut meat. Also, keep separate cutting boards for meat and fish, and be sure to thoroughly wash all vegetables and fruit.

As for removing parasites from the body, Dr. Chaitow, author of *Candida Albicans*, has had an 80 percent success rate with CRC patients by using high-dosage probiotic supplements. He recommends the three probiotic supplements, *Lactobacillus acidophilus*, *Lactobacillus bulgaricus*, and bifidobacteria. The treatment generally lasts between eight and twelve weeks. Another natural way to rid the body of parasites is with citrus seed extract, which is frequently used in other countries to treat parasitic infections.

Mercury-Silver Fillings: Possible Toxins in Your Mouth

Although mercury-silver dental amalgam has been extensively studied and considered safe for many years, there is growing concern and disturbing evidence that mercury-silver dental amalgam fillings are toxic to the body and disruptive to the immune system. Silver fillings, which are put in about two hundred million teeth a year, contain a mixture of silver, zinc, tin, copper, and usually 50 percent mercury. Germany has banned the sale and manufacture of amalgams since 1992, and Sweden has promised to ban amalgams as soon as a safe substitute can be found. Until a substitute is found the Swedish government pays 50 percent of the amalgam removal cost.

The ADA (American Dental Association) reports that mercury amalgam fillings are not dangerous except to a small number of people who have severe allergic reactions to mercury. In a summary of its position on mercury amalgams (which has long been challenged by an increasing number of dentists), the ADA has this to say:

> Dental amalgam has an indisputable safety record and has been extensively reviewed. The U.S. Public Health Service issued a report in 1993 stating there is no health reason not to use amalgam, except in the extremely rare case of the patient who is allergic to a component of amalgam. This supports the findings of the Food and Drug Administration (FDA), the National Institutes of Health Technology Assessment Conference and the National Institutes of Dental Research (NIDR) that dental amalgam is a safe and effective restorative material. In addition, in 1991, *Consumer Reports* noted that 'given their solid track record . . . amalgam fillings are still your best bet.'

According to the ADA, when mercury amalgams are in place in the mouth, they harden and do not release mercury vapors. However, a study published in the *Journal of Dental Research* in September 1981 found people with mercury amalgams in their mouths had mercury vapors in their mouths at levels 15,600 percent higher than people who did not have mercury amalgams.

Dentists follow strict procedures when storing and handling mercury amalgams, and the ADA routinely conducts annual screenings to determine whether or not their dentists test positively for dangerously high levels of mercury. In 1988, the Environmental Protection Agency (EPA) declared scrap dental amalgam a *hazardous waste*, which means it can't be put in a landfill, thrown out with regular trash, or buried in the ground.

Although in the past decade there has been a very public controversy about the safety of such fillings, this debate is not new. Dentists have been protesting mercury amalgam fillings since their first use in 1833. At that time increased sugar consumption was causing widespread tooth decay, and an affordable substance for filling teeth was needed because gold was too expensive. Mercury amalgam fillings were not introduced by professional dentists, but by dental entrepreneurs. They were strongly protested by licensed dentists. Dr. Lorenzani explains in her detailed description of the dangers of mercury in the body:

> Professional dentists rose in outrage to protest the use of a compound they claimed was poisonous and would result in gum disease and other ills. The American Society of Dental Surgeons denounced silver-mercury fillings as 'hurtful both to the tooth and all parts of the mouth.' Members pledged not to use mercury in treating their patients. Dictates of principle also included principles of economics. More and more dentists quietly turned to mercury amalgams as an affordable alternative to gold. As time went on, these dentists organized to argue that mercury fillings were actually safe as well as inexpensive.

Just how toxic is mercury to the body? Mercury is in fact considered to be more toxic than arsenic. If mercury reaches the bloodstream, it will be transported throughout the body, where it has different effects on the organs of the body. Studies on animals and humans have shown that when mercury comes in contact with blood, it damages the cells that normally protect us from disease. Mercury also causes structural damage in the brain and alters brain chemistry. When mercury reaches the heart via the bloodstream, it is shown capable of interfering with normal cardiac functions. Mercury also destroys kidney cells and causes protein to be lost from the body via urine. Enormous amounts of mercury (often more than can be found in mercury amalgams) have also been shown to cause tremors, loss of vision and hearing, and impaired muscle coordination.

Given what we know about mercury, there seems to be every reason to worry about using it as a dental filling. Not only do we know mercury is harmful to the body even in small doses, but its safety as a dental filling has never been established. Recent evidence shows that when placed into the body in the form of dental amalgams, mercury is released into the body. According to Dr. Lorenzani, "There is an impressive and steadily increasing collection of scientific research showing that the mercury in dental fillings leaks into the teeth, gums, and air in the mouth. Then it may be swallowed, inhaled, and absorbed into the bloodstream." Common symptoms associated with mercury amalgam fillings include headaches, fatigue, muscle and joint pains, central nervous system disorders, and a variety of other seemingly unexplainable problems.

Drs. Trowbridge and Walker, authors of *The Yeast Syndrome*, emphasize the dangers of mercury amalgam fillings and strongly suggest that CRC patients have their fillings replaced with safer substances. They point out that clinical reports confirm that some patients suffering with disorders of the Candida syndrome fail to get well on the usual antifungal therapy alone, although they do recover after the source of mercury intoxication is eliminated. According to Drs. Trowbridge and Walker, the use of mercury as a dental filling is widespread. In 1980 alone, American dentists used two hundred thousand pounds of mercury for fillings in teeth. In 1985 this amount increased to three hundred thousand pounds.

On the bright side, many more dentists have recently begun questioning the use of mercury as a dental filling. According to a 1990 survey, 6 percent of dentists did not use mercury amalgams in their dental practice, and 39 percent of dentists said they were either "concerned" or "highly concerned" about the safety of mercury as a dental filling material.

Although mercury amalgam dental fillings don't cause health problems for everyone, they still contribute to our toxic load, which in turn affects our resistance to infection. Mercury can negatively affect our immune systems, especially immune systems of people who are already ill. For a list of mercury-free dentists in your area, send a business-sized, self-addressed stamped envelope to the Foundation for Toxic-Free Dentistry, P.O. Box 608010, Orlando, FL, 32860.

For more information on mercury amalgam fillings, contact the Environmental Dental Association at 9974 Scripps Ranch Blvd., Suite 36, San Diego, CA, 92131, (800) 388-8124. Another source for information is the Huggins Diagnostic Center, 5080 List Dr., Colorado Springs, CO, 80919, (800) 331-2303. If you do decide to have your mercury amalgam fillings removed, be sure to go to a dentist who has been specially trained in sequential mercury amalgam dental filling removal.

Although CRC can take months or even years of careful health monitoring, the majority of patients who keep working on their health do succeed. Don't forget that the key to recovering from CRC is to stimulate your body's own immune defenses so they can take care of the problems from within. Also remember to have patience with yourself and your health, because a full recovery takes time.

—13—

Treatments for Vaginal Infections

Vaginitis must cause more unhappiness on earth than any other gynecologic disease. In addition to the many physical and emotional problems associated with vaginitis, the economic loss involved is of astronomical proportions.
—Herman Gardner in *Benign Diseases of the Vulva and Vagina*

Vaginitis, an inflammation or infection of the vagina, is both a commonly reported symptom of CRC and a problem an estimated 75 percent of women have at least once in their lives. In the U.S. alone, over twenty-two million women have vaginitis every year. In 1990 alone, sales for prescription medications for vaginal infections reached $220 million, and sales for over-the-counter (OTC) vaginal medications were expected to reach over $400 million within five years. Despite the obvious problem women have with vaginal infections, they continue to be trivialized by some physicians as "minor feminine irritation."

Many women with CRC have persistent vaginal problems and have difficulty relieving their discomfort. Women with CRC have a high incidence of vaginal problems because the same impaired immune defenses that made them susceptible to CRC also fail to protect them when Candida gets the upper hand in the ever-present war between the microorganisms in the vagina.

The term *vaginitis* describes any and all vaginal infections, yeast infections, and inflammations. The term *yeast infection* is often used to describe a Candidal vaginal infection. The general symptoms of vaginitis are vaginal burning, itching, a foul odor, and discharge. The area surrounding the vagina may become red, feel irritated, and appear sore. Vulvitis, inflammation of the vulva, often accompanies vaginal infections and responds well to the same treatments for vaginitis.

Women are especially susceptible to vaginal problems during their menstrual cycles, when they are pregnant, if they take birth control pills (which simulate pregnancy), or if they have to take steroids or antibiotics. Other things that can cause vaginitis include a high-sugar diet, sexual intercourse (Candida can be sexually transmitted), use of spermicides, frequent sexual intercourse (semen alters the pH level of the vagina), diabetes, a chemical irritant, emotional stress, excessive douching, and a vitamin B deficiency. Whatever the initial trigger, the result is a change in the acidity of the vagina that renders the patient susceptible to an infection. As with CRC, the problem is not the Candida organism, which cannot harm a healthy individual, the problem is whatever weakened the immune system in the first place.

The vagina is constantly changing. It's affected by many things, including your diet, menstrual cycle, any medications you may be taking, and sexual arousal. Some discharge and odor are perfectly normal. All women secrete mucus and moisture from the membranes that line the vagina. This discharge has various appearances and can be clear or slightly milky and even clumpy like cottage cheese. When dry, the discharge is often yellow. Normal vaginal discharges do not have a foul odor and do not irritate the vagina or vulva. Normal discharges also do not cause burning or itching.

You and Your Gynecologist: Getting the Care You Need

If you have any doubts about a vaginal infection, go to your gynecologist immediately. Although vaginal infections aren't life-threatening, you need to be very careful about your health while you have CRC and even after you have it under control. A vaginal infection could indicate anything from an internal infection to a sexually transmitted disease. For example, if you have an intrauterine device (IUD), an abnormal vaginal problem or discharge could indicate an infection in your uterus. Here are some general guidelines that will help you decide when it's time to go to your doctor:

- If this is your first vaginal infection or discharge.
- If your vaginitis symptoms recur within a two-month time period.
- If you have a new sexual partner, you have several sexual partners, or if your sexual partner has several sexual partners. You could be at risk for sexually transmitted infections.

- If you are pregnant. Both trichomonas vaginitis and bacterial vaginosis can seriously complicate pregnancy, and a Candidal infection can be passed to the baby via the birth process.

- If you are familiar with Candidal vaginal infections and what you have seems to be something other than a simple Candidal vaginal infection. If you suspect you have trichomoniasis or a bacterial infection, go to your gynecologist immediately to get the correct prescription medications and be thoroughly examined and tested for gonorrhea or other sexually transmitted diseases.

- If you are familiar with Candidal vaginal infections and believe you have a Candidal vaginal infection, yet the usual medications and remedies aren't working.

- If your symptoms persist after three to four days, if they get worse, or if they occur along with severe pain, heavy bleeding, or fever. In this case, you should immediately go to your gynecologist, urgent care center, or emergency room.

It is important for your physician to do a thorough examination and to take a vaginal discharge or infection seriously. The only exception might be if your present infection is something you and your physician are familiar with and have treated previously, but even then a pelvic exam should be performed. Your physician should take your complete medical history, perform a pelvic exam, and then perform several tests to help determine what caused the infection. Although many physicians still use a Pap smear, recent research has shown that Pap smears are unreliable as a diagnostic tool for vaginal infections and test positive in only 25 percent of the cases studied. Your physician may still want to perform a Pap smear to test for cervical cancer, and this is a good idea if you haven't had one done recently. The tests your physician performs *must* include a thorough microscopic examination of a sample taken from the vaginal wall to test for Candida, trichomonas, and bacterial vaginosis. Clinical signs and symptoms and a culture that positively tests for Candida are not enough. Since they are all normal inhabitants of the vagina, the presence or absence of Candida, bacteria, or trichomonas does not necessarily indicate that your infection is specifically caused by these organisms.

The tests your physician performs will depend on several things, including whether he or she has ever examined you before, how long it has been since you have had routine tests done, and what he or she finds during the pelvic exam. If you are sexually active, have an abnormal discharge, and haven't been tested recently, you should be tested for gonorrhea and other diseases. Gonorrhea frequently causes infections in the cervix that can lead to infertility. As *Every Woman's Health*, edited by Helene MacLean, notes, "Because there are so many different organisms and conditions that may result in vaginitis, it is necessary to find the cause by physical examination, cultures, and microscopic examination of the vaginal discharge before attempting treatment. Because the urethra and bladder are so close to the vulva and vagina, an infection in one area may cause symptoms in the other, making diagnosis difficult."

Despite the obviously large problem vaginal infections are for women everywhere, they are not taken seriously by many practicing physicians. This attitude is reflected in the medical care given to women with vaginitis. As Jack D. Sobel, M.D., editor of *Vulvovaginal Infections*, writes in the preface of his book:

> Vaginitis as a distinct clinical entity enjoys a strikingly low order of priority in the education of residents in the various medical disciplines that ultimately provide primary or secondary level care for women. Since no one dies of vaginitis and rarely are patients hospitalized with cervicitis or vaginitis, lower genital tract infections are viewed by most clinicians as being of nuisance value only.

Dr. Sobel also writes that this disturbing but prevalent attitude is often translated into inadequate clinical and diagnostic efforts to reach the appropriate diagnosis. Because vaginitis isn't taken seriously by many physicians, they treat women empirically, which means their diagnosis is based on what they find during the pelvic exam or based on their experiences with other female patients. Their diagnosis is frequently not based on test results or other information from patients.

Because the diagnosis may or may not be accurate and isn't customized to the patient, the medicines prescribed may or may not work and the infection may or may not heal. More importantly, a bacterial or other serious infection may be missed. In an essay on Candidal vulvovaginitis in *Vulvovaginal Infections*, Dr. Sobel reports that at the Detroit Medical Center Candida Vaginitis Clinic, more than 80 percent of incalcitrant or recurrent Candidal vaginitis infections were found to have been caused by something other than Candidal vaginitis. A 1991 article in the *American Journal of Obstetrics and Gynecology* by Leonard J. Cibley, M.D., and Laurence J. Cibley, M.D., also confirms the inaccuracy of a physician's visual diagnosis. The authors write, "We challenged the accuracy of the 'eyeball' diagnosis at the 1985 national meeting of the American College of Obstetricians and Gynecologists. In a scientific exhibit, after viewing a series of slides, participants were asked to register a diagnosis based solely on color, consistency, and physical characteristics. The average score of those physicians was 30 percent."

Because vaginal infections aren't taken seriously, either by the educational institutions that shape the minds and determine the priorities of budding physicians, or by most practicing doctors, it is up to you to make sure you get the attention and care you need and deserve. If you suspect your infection is not Candida-related, insist that your gynecologist give your problem the time and seriousness it deserves by doing the appropriate tests. If your physician disparages you or your concerns about your health, find another physician. Caring and professional doctors do not need to be reminded of their responsibilities and would not view helping you as an inconvenience or a waste of their time.

In January 1991, miconazole (Monistat) and clotrimazole (Gyne-Lotrimin) were approved by the Food and Drug Administration (FDA) as nonprescription therapies for Candidal vaginitis. This decision brought nationwide attention to the problem of yeast infections and was welcomed by many women as a convenient and easy way to treat their vaginitis. Although many physicians applauded the FDA's decision in helping patients gain immediate access to treatment, others were justifiably concerned that a certain percentage of women might not get the medical care they need. By treating their own vaginal infections, some women may miss a mixed infection or misdiagnose their problem as Candida-related when it is actually bacterial vaginosis or trichomonas vaginitis. A self-misdiagnosis would keep women from getting the correct treatment. Physicians are also concerned that over-the-counter treatments for vaginitis will encourage women to avoid their gynecologists. Before over-the-counter medications were available, a vaginal infection often prompted women to visit their physicians, who performed routine exams and basic preventative gynecological health care in addition to treating the infection. Nonprescription medications are quick and convenient, but they should not be used as a way to avoid regular appointments with your gynecologist or as a substitute for necessary medical care. It is extremely important to visit your gynecologist yearly (or more often if you have problems or health concerns).

If you have Candidal vaginal infections from time to time and are able to successfully treat them with nonprescription medications and natural treatments, you probably do not need to go to your gynecologist. However, if you have any doubts about the seriousness of a vaginal infection, or have difficulty with recurring infections or infections that do not respond to treatment, do not hesitate to consult a doctor.

General Treatment Guidelines and Remedies for All Vaginal Infections

Whatever kind of vaginitis you have, all vaginal infections come with predictable symptoms, including burning, itching, soreness, discharge, and a foul odor. Be sure to not scratch the infected area and to keep your vagina as clean as possible.

For vaginal problems, many women rely on a combination of prescription medication and nonprescription remedies that include medical creams, suppositories, and alternative treatments. Perhaps the easiest and most important natural therapy you can use to prevent infections and to help heal yourself when you have an infection is the use of *Lactobacillus acidophilus*. These microorganisms, which destroy Candida, are normally present in the bowel and vagina. Increasing the amount of acidophilus in your body, either by eating fresh, homemade yogurt or by taking acidophilus supplements, will also help restore the flora in your vagina and the rest of your body. The following yogurt/lactobacillus remedy has been helpful to hundreds of Dr. Sehnert's patients: mix one tablespoon of plain yogurt with the powder from two capsules of acidophilus. Stir well and apply it to a fresh tampon. Insert it into the vagina at bedtime and leave it in all night. Do this for three consecutive nights.

Recent research has indicated that douching pushes bacteria from the vagina into the uterus and can lead to pelvic inflammatory disease (PID). Because of this, it is a good idea to avoid douching unless your physician recommends otherwise. Many women find taking sitz baths helpful in preventing infections and relieving vaginal itching. Sitz baths are a safe alternative to douching. A vinegar sitz bath (made with pure apple cider vinegar) helps restore the natural pH of the vagina and can be prepared by adding one-half cup of vinegar to warm, shallow water in your bath tub. If your vagina has the correct pH balance the area is less receptive to Candida overgrowth. A salt sitz bath, which can help relieve itching, can be prepared by adding about one-half cup of salt (enough to make the water taste a little salty) to a warm, shallow bath. For best results sit in the bath with your knees apart for about twenty minutes or until the water cools. Another way to relieve genital itching is to apply vitamin E oil to the area. Even though vitamin E oil is sold in small jars, it is more sanitary to prick a capsule. Aloe vera gel and calendula cream can also be used to relieve vaginal itching and soreness and can be applied directly to the affected area or put on a sanitary pad.

Garlic, which specifically inhibits yeast growth, is an important supplement to take when you are having vaginal problems and can be particularly helpful in suppository form. Taking vitamins, especially vitamin C, will help boost your immunity. Other nutrients you may find helpful are yeast-free vitamin B complex, vitamin B_6, vitamin A, and vitamin E. Vitamin D with added calcium and magnesium will help the body fight infection and repair damage caused by Candida infection.

In *A Woman's Guide to Yeast Infections*, Naomi Baumslag, M.D., and Dia L. Michels recommend boric acid suppositories as a safe and inexpensive treatment for vaginal infections. Several studies have also shown boric acid suppositories to be helpful in preventing recurrent infections. Boric acid is a colorless and odorless powder that is usually used as an antiseptic. It can be very toxic and lead to death if ingested or used improperly, and is for external use only. Be very careful to keep and store boric acid away from children.

Boric acid is found in many personal-care products, including skin ointments, eye drops, mouthwashes, and hemorrhoidal suppositories. The only known side effect from boric acid suppositories is a minimal watery discharge during treatment. You can also use boric acid ointment twice daily for outer vaginal and vulvar itching, redness, and swelling. You can make your own boric acid suppositories from empty gelatin capsules and boric acid powder (not crystals), both available at your local pharmacy. The powder should be located in the eye care section of the store, and you should look for size 0 or 00 gelatin capsules. Insert one prepared capsule into your vagina every morning and evening for ten to fourteen days. Do not use boric acid suppositories if you have vaginal cuts, abrasions, or open vaginal or cervical sores.

Three Different Types of Vaginal Infections and Specific Treatments

The three major types of vaginitis are Candidal vaginitis, trichomonas vaginitis, and bacterial vaginosis. The term *vaginosis* is used instead of *vaginitis* to describe a bacterial infection because *vaginitis* signifies an inflammation, and bacterial infections are not accompanied by inflammation. Vaginitis can also be caused by nonspecific and often chemical irritants, including products such as douches, deodorants, sprays, tampons, maxi pads, spermicides, perfumed soaps, bubble baths or oils, or a foreign body in your vagina such as a lost or forgotten tampon. Many women are told by physicians that they have recurrent vaginitis when in fact they are just very sensitive or allergic to an irritant around them. General vaginitis symptoms include inflammation, itching, and a discharge. When vaginitis has been caused by a chemical irritant, it will subside with medication and will not reoccur unless the irritant comes in contact with the vagina again.

Although they should be aware of the other types of vaginal infections, women with CRC seem to predominantly have problems with Candidal vaginitis because of the Candida growth within their bodies. However, just because you have always had Candidal vaginal infections doesn't mean that every infection you get will be Candida-related. If you have unprotected sexual intercourse, you may be at risk for trichomonas vaginitis and bacterial vaginosis.

As mentioned earlier in this chapter, Candida can be sexually transmitted, and in fact the Centers for Disease Control (CDC) classifies Candidal vaginitis as a venereal disease, partially for record-keeping purposes. Candidal infections can, and often are, passed back and forth between male and female partners. Recent research shows that of the patients surveyed, 15 percent have noticed that Candida has been transmitted back and forth between themselves and their partners. In 1985, Dr. Sobel found that the male sexual partners of women with yeast infections are four times more likely to have penile colonization than partners of women without vaginal infections. Penile colonization means that Candida is present in significant amounts on the penis. It can be asymptomatic, which means it is harmless to the carrier, but remains a possible source of reinfection to the woman. When symptoms, such as penile itching, dryness, redness, inflammation, and red spots on the penis are present, the Candidal infection is called Candida balanoposthitis or Candida balanitis. The most common treatments for male partners is caprylic acid supplements (available in health food stores), nystatin, and oral antifungal drugs. If you suspect that you and your partner are transmitting Candida between one another, bring your partner to the physician with you.

Candidal Vaginitis
A vaginal infection caused by Candida has several classic symptoms, which include severe itching, irritation, soreness, redness in the vaginal and/or vulval area, bleeding upon urination, pain or discomfort during intercourse, abdominal pain, and sometimes vaginal bleeding. Another common symptom is a thick white discharge, which may have a thin consistency, but often has the consistency of cottage cheese.

Candida organisms are usually kept in check by other organisms that inhabit the vagina, including lactobacilli. Candidal vaginal infections, often called yeast infections, occur when something alters the delicate balance between the organisms in the vagina and the yeast growth gets out of control. The overgrowth of yeast causes an inflammatory response along the walls of the vagina, which leads to the common symptoms of this vaginal infection.

Candidal vaginal infections are extremely common. An estimated 75 percent of women will experience at least one Candidal vaginitis infection during their childbearing years. Forty to 50 percent of women will experience a second incident. A small amount of adult women, less than 5 percent, experience recurrent and sometimes difficult-to-treat episodes of Candidal vaginitis. Vaginitis accounts for more than ten million office visits every year and is the most common reason a woman visits her obstetrician-gynecologist.

In his essay on Candida vulvovaginitis in *Vulvovaginal Infections,* Dr. Sobel makes the point that an estimated 15 to 25 percent of non-pregnant premenopausal women have asymptomatic colonization, sometimes for months at a time. This means that they have significant amounts of Candida in their vagina, but do not have symptoms of a Candidal infection. For an infection or problem to arise, something must happen to either initiate colonization and/or change the colonization to vaginitis.

Sometimes the yeast infection has a discernible cause, but infections often happen for no apparent reason. Symptomatic vaginitis tends to develop when a combination of circumstances occur. Certain factors increase the ability of Candida to cause disease, or the natural defensive mechanisms fail to protect the body. As might be expected, women with CRC frequently have vaginal problems and infections, in part because their immune systems have difficulty clearing their bodies of the unwelcome visitor. Many factors are capable of altering the balance between the organisms in the vagina and triggering an infection.

Dr. Sobel lists eight known factors that are capable of initiating both asymptomatic colonization and symptomatic vaginitis, and these factors can increase the virulence of Candida and suppress natural bodily defense mechanisms. They are pregnancy, uncontrolled diabetes mellitus, high-estrogen-containing oral contraceptives, corticosteroid therapy, tight-fitting synthetic underclothing, antibiotic therapy (both oral/systemic and topical/local), increased frequency of coitus (semen alters the pH level of the vagina), and candy binges. Dr. Sobel notes that two of the eight factors, the increased frequency of coitus and candy binges, are associated only with symptomatic vaginitis. According to Dr. Sobel, these factors alter the vaginal microenvironment, which leads to Candida multiplication and germination, and to the changing of the microenvironment from one that didn't encourage Candida growth to one that does. The environment is changed in a number of ways: more nutrients exist for Candida while the naturally restraining mechanisms Dr. Sobel describes as "biologic brakes," supplied by the bacterial flora of the body and the mucosal immune system, are eliminated.

Dr. Sobel's observations and research are important to note because the critical issue about vaginal infections isn't that especially virulent strains of Candida exist, or that better medicines need to be developed. The issue is that you, the host, play an important part in the development of vaginitis. Treating your vaginitis with oral or topical medications is necessary and important, but when possible, you need to avoid those factors (listed earlier) that increase your chances of developing symptomatic vaginitis.

Since Candidal vaginitis can be sexually transmitted between male and female partners, be sure to ask your physician if your partner should be treated as well as yourself. Many physicians feel men should be treated simultaneously, especially in the case of difficult-to-treat infections or recurrent infections.

When helping your physician select a treatment regimen, it is important to determine whether you have infrequent or recurrent vaginitis. The distinction between the two types of infections is important because it helps determine the length of time you will need to take medications and whether or not a maintenance regimen is necessary for you. Women with infrequent infections have three or less a year. Women with four or more infections during a one-year period have recurrent Candidal vaginitis. These distinctions are important because they will help you and your doctor best decide how to effectively treat your infections. A maintenance regimen to help prevent infections may be in your best interest. Many women with CRC report having vaginal infections from time to time until they get their CRC under control.

For most women, infrequent infections can be successfully treated with natural remedies, including nonprescription creams or suppositories, and short treatment regimens of prescribed medicine. If you have recurrent infections, you will have to follow a longer treatment regimen to be sure the infection has been cured or subdued as much as possible. You also need to anticipate infections and to use medications to help keep them from occurring whenever possible. No matter what kind of infection you have, if you are pregnant your physician will advise you to follow a longer treatment regimen. Episodes of Candidal vaginitis are extremely common during pregnancy and the response to treatment is often slower and recurrences more likely to happen.

Because many patients don't complete the entire regimen of medication and because many patients prefer oral treatment over topical treatment, there have been many changes in the vaginitis treatments available. A wider variety of choices are now available, including new oral medications and topical medications with increased dosages and shorter treatment regimens. In clinical studies, shortened treatment regimens have been found to be as effective for patients with mild or moderate infections as longer treatment regimens. Although shortened regimens are good for some patients, women with severe vaginal infections or a history of such infections should be given prolonged regimens.

Although more studies need to be conducted, shortened treatment regimens and antifungal drugs that do not act against different types of Candida may be responsible for the increase in vaginal infections caused by Candida species other than *Candida albicans*. Although the medications used in the shortened treatment regimens suppress *Candida albicans*, many do not act against non-albicans Candida species. A 1992 article in the *Journal of Clinical Pharmacology* states that shortened treatment regimens may imbalance vaginal microflora and facilitate the overgrowth of other Candida species. Infections by non-albicans species of Candida have more than doubled from the 1970s to the 1980s, rising from 9.9 percent to 21.3 percent. Two of the top offenders are *Candida tropicalis* and *Candida glabrata*. Because vaginal infections by non-albicans species are increasing, drugs that act against non-albicans strains of Candida are being more widely used, and more drugs that kill these strains need to be developed.

The introduction of shorter regimens is also a way pharmaceutical companies can compete for patient dollars. Single-dose regimens are not cheaper than longer regimens; pharmaceutical companies have priced them the same as longer conventional therapies. Dr. Sobel makes several key points on this subject in a 1994 article in the *Journal of the American Academy of Dermatology*:

> Although justified on the basis of convenience and improved compliance, these new regimens have also been introduced to provide a marketing edge for one therapeutically equivalent agent over another. Testing the efficacy of short, often single-dose courses has not been subject to the same careful and thorough scrutiny as conventional five- to seven-day regimens; neither are these shorter courses less expensive. Nevertheless, single-dose therapy by any route is effective in mild-to-moderate disease and no less so than conventional therapy.

The following chart is a general guide to the usual drugs, dosages, and treatment regimens for Candidal vaginal infections. This chart is a guide only. As more research is done, this information could change, so your final source for information should be your physician and the treatment information that accompanies your medication.

THERAPIES FOR VAGINAL CANDIDAL INFECTIONS

Drug	Formulation	Dosage
Butoconazole (Femstat)	2% cream	5g at bedtime for 3 days
Clotrimazole (Gyne-Lotrimin)	1% cream	5g at bedtime for 7 to 14 days
Mycelex	10% cream	5g single application
	100mg vaginal tablet	1 tablet at bedtime for 7 days
	100mg vaginal tablet	2 tablets at bedtime for 3 days
	500mg vaginal tablet	1 tablet once
Econazole	150mg vaginal tablet	1 tablet at bedtime for 3 days
Fenticonazole	2% cream	5g at bedtime for 7 days
Fluconazole (Diflucan)	Oral tablet	150mg once
Itraconazole	100mg tablet	200mg orally for 3 days
Ketoconazole (Nizerol)	200mg tablet	400mg orally for 5 days
Miconazole (Monistat)	2% cream	5g at bedtime for 7 days
	100mg vaginal suppository	1 suppository at bedtime for 7 days
	200mg vaginal suppository	1 suppository at bedtime for 3 days
	1,200mg vaginal suppository	1 suppository once
Nystatin (Micostatin, Nilstat)	100,000-unit tablet	1 tablet at bedtime for 14 days
Terconazole	2% cream	5g at bedtime for 3 days
Tioconazole	2% cream	5g at bedtime for 3 days
	6.5% cream	5g at bedtime once

Adapted with permission from *Vulvovaginal Infections*

Of the medicines listed above, all but nystatin belong to the azole family of drugs described in chapter 11. Research done on the topical forms of the azoles used to treat vaginitis has shown that they have an 80 to 90 percent cure rate. Although these numbers are encouraging, Naomi Baumslag, M.D., and Dia L. Michels write in *A Woman's Guide to Yeast Infections*, "this [percentage] is actually fairly low when you consider we are dealing with a local treatment of a condition involving one single pathogen at an accessible site."

In comparative clinical tests, none of the individual azole drugs appears to be superior in cure rates, although several appear to offer other important advantages that relate to recurrent cases of Candidal vaginitis. For instance, terconazole has a wide range of activity against not only *Candida albicans,* but other Candida strains. This ability makes it ideal for women whose vaginal infections may not be caused specifically by *Candida albicans* and for those who have recurrent infections that are resistant to other treatments.

Candida albicans is not the only strain of Candida capable of causing vaginal infections. As mentioned earlier, other strains are being increasingly held responsible for vaginal infections. To date there is no reason to believe the other strains of Candida are more virulent than *Candida albicans,* although research has indicated that not all the azole drugs are equally effective against different strains of Candida. A 1991 article in the *American Journal of Obstetrics and Gynecology* reports that two strains of the Candida family, *Candida tropicalis* and *Candida glabrata,* are ten times less sensitive than *Candida albicans* to miconazole (Monistat). Another yeast, called Rhodotorula, is also insensitive to miconazole.

Two new advantageous drugs are the oral forms of itraconazole (Sporanox) and fluconazole (Diflucan). Research has shown that these two drugs are extremely effective in eliminating the rectal carriage of the Candida species and therefore may help prevent recurrent infections. If your physician prescribes itraconazole, *be sure not to take it with Seldane or Hismanal.* Patients who have taken itraconazole with these two drugs have had serious health problems. Fluconazole should not be taken with anticoagulants, antidiabetic drugs, some antihistamines (such as Hismanal), ulcer medications (including Tagamet), Phenytoin, cyclosporine, hydrochlorothiazide, and rifampin.

Always let your doctor and pharmacist know your medication history and any reactions or sensitivities you have had to other drugs, both prescription and nonprescription. If you have ever had a reaction or a sensitivity to an azole drug, you should not take another azole drug. Most topical therapies for vaginal Candidal infections, including the azoles, have very few side effects, although the initial topical application may be uncomfortable and cause a burning sensation. In a 1990 article published in the *Journal of the American Academy of Dermatology,* Dr. Sobel explains that a burning sensation upon application of an imidazole cream represents a local irritant reaction rather than an allergic reaction. Often the ingredients in the cream and not the actual antifungal medication are responsible. Dr. Sobel reports that topical miconazole and tioconazole are generally found to be associated with local burning symptoms, while terconazole seems to have the fewest local side effects.

It is important for you to work closely with your physician so she can best select the treatment and treatment regimen that will best help you cure your vaginitis. In his 1990 article in the *Journal of the American Academy of Dermatology*, Dr. Sobel lists several factors your physician will need to take into account before selecting your medication, the form of your medication, and the duration of your treatment. These factors can be divided into two categories: the physical and clinical diagnosis of this episode of vaginitis, and the information you give your physician about your present and past vaginal infections. The physical and clinical information your physician will take into consideration will include the severity of the signs and symptoms of your present attack, the anatomic distribution of the inflammation, the possibility of a mixed infection, the possibility of resistant microorganisms, whether or not you are pregnant, and your physician's impression of your ability to follow a prescribed regimen. Unless your physician gives you other instructions, always follow the entire prescribed regimen for Candidal vaginitis and all other types of vaginitis to help prevent the infection from returning.

The information your physician will need you to provide includes your history of infections, your good and bad experiences with other medications, and how long you have had your present vaginal infection. The growing number of options for treating Candidal vaginitis has left some doctors confused as to what type and form of medication may be best for each patient. Because of the relatively equal cure rate of the newer medications available, your doctor's choice will be based on many factors, including his or her experiences with the individual medications, which medication seems to best apply to your situation, and the cost of the medication (especially if the cost isn't covered by health insurance). You can help your physician by telling him or her if you have a preference for an oral or topical form of medicine and if you are more likely to complete a short treatment regimen.

Trichomonas Vaginitis

The symptoms of trichomonas vaginitis, also known as trich, are itching or vaginal irritation, which often worsens after the menstrual cycle; a burning sensation upon urination; and frequent urination. Another symptom is a thin, sometimes frothy, foul-smelling yellow-green discharge that may or may not be mixed with blood.

Trichomonas vaginitis is caused by *Trichomonas vaginalis*, a one-celled organism that can live in the urethra and prostate of men, and the urethra, bladder, vagina, and cervix of women. Trichomonas affects an estimated three million women every year. Trichomonas vaginitis is often diagnosed through a clinical test of the discharge. Trichomonas can be very serious and can cause cystitis, an inflammation of the bladder. Women who get this very uncomfortable disease are almost always sexually active, and the disease is often sexually transmitted. Because of this, it is technically classified as a venereal disease. Men who carry the Trichomonas organism or have trichomoniasis may have a slight discharge from their penis or burning upon urination.

Trichomonas vaginitis is usually treated with metronidazole (Flagyl and Protostat), an antiprotozal/antibacterial that is the only medication found to have a significant cure rate. The treatment regimen usually lasts for one week. It is very important that you take all the medicine and that you take acidophilus supplements before, during, and after taking metronidazole. Recent studies have also shown that a single oral dose (determined by your physician) is very effective and can have fewer side effects.

Metronidazole can have serious side effects, including seizures and tingling or numbness in hands, arms, feet, and legs. Less serious but frequently reported side effects include nausea, diarrhea, abdominal cramps, constipation, upset stomach, vomiting, and headaches. A small percentage of women find that when taking metronidazole their tongues feel furry, they have a strange taste in their mouths, and their urine becomes dark. People taking metronidazole should also strictly avoid alcohol, both while taking the medication and for twenty-four hours after their last dose. Also be sure to avoid nonprescription medications that contain alcohol, such as cough syrups and cold preparations. Metronidazole should also be taken with a meal. To prevent reinfection, it is important that sexual partners of women with trichomonas vaginitis be treated whether or not they show symptoms. As with all medications, be sure your physician knows what medications you are taking, both prescription and nonprescription, so drug interactions can be avoided.

The treatment of trichomonas vaginitis during pregnancy can be difficult because metronidazole is the only effective drug available, and women who are pregnant (particularly in their first trimester) or nursing a child should not take metronidazole. If you are pregnant, your physician will probably prescribe 100mg clotrimazole suppositories for two weeks. This treatment regimen has a 50 percent cure rate. Trichomonas vaginitis can complicate pregnancy, so if you are pregnant you should immediately see your physician. According to a 1991 article in the *American Journal of Obstetrics and Gynecology*, a recent study has shown that the carriage of the trichomonas organism is independently associated with low-birth weight infants and premature rupture of fetal membranes. It is unknown whether the actual organism is responsible, or if the possible complications are from the flora associated with the other sexually transmitted diseases that often accompany trichomonas vaginitis.

Bacterial Vaginosis

The two typical symptoms of bacterial vaginosis are an increased discharge, which can sometimes range in color from white to grayish and watery, and a very foul, often fishy, odor. Women with bacterial vaginosis may not have symptoms other than a fishy odor and do not usually report inflammation as a symptom. If you have additional symptoms, you may have a mixed infection. In fact, bacterial vaginosis often coexists with trichomonas vaginitis. Your gynecologist can perform a lab test to determine if you have bacterial vaginosis.

Bacterial vaginosis is caused by bacteria, often *Gardnerella vaginalis*, which has most likely been sexually transmitted or has found its way from your anus to your vagina. Bacterial vaginosis is the most prevalent infectious cause of vaginitis. Confirmation that you have certain kinds of bacteria in your vagina does not prove you have bacterial vaginosis. Since Gardnerella is found in 40 to 50 percent of women who do not have vaginitis, its presence or the presence of any kind of bacteria does not necessarily indicate a diagnosis of bacterial vaginosis. As David A. Eschenbach, M.D., writes in his essay in *Vulvovaginal Infections*, "Perhaps it is the increased concentration of bacteria that characterizes BV [bacterial vaginosis] rather than an increased prevalence of organisms, although both do occur. Normal concentrations of bacteria in the vagina (usually 10^5 organisms/mL of vaginal fluid) increase to 10^{8-9} organisms/mL in women with BV."

Unfortunately, more research needs to be done on bacterial vaginosis because many aspects of the disease are not clear. Facts yet to be determined include whether or not it is sexually transmitted; the male sexual partner's role in bacterial vaginosis; and nonsexual risk factors. As Dr. Eschenbach writes, "Treating male partners with metronidazole has no effect on the recurrence of BV in women. The male role is further complicated by the possibility that uncircumcised men may be a factor in the development of BV. Other nonsexual risk factors have been found as well. IUDs appear to increase the risk of infection. Frequency of intercourse, oral or rectal sexual contact, douching, tampon use, and antibiotics do not seem to be related to BV."

If you do have bacterial vaginosis, your physician will probably have to prescribe an antibiotic, so be prepared to take acidophilus supplements and to follow the other natural remedies described in this chapter. Metronidazole (Flagyl and Protostat), which is also used to treat trichomonas vaginitis, is the most effective drug available to treat bacterial vaginosis. A seven-day course of metronidazole is recommended; single-dose regimens have been shown to not be effective. It is uncertain whether or not treating sexual partners of women with bacterial vaginosis prevents relapses of the disease. The side effects of metronidazole are discussed in the section on trichomonas vaginitis. Although there have not yet been any published reports on cephalexin (Keflex), an antibiotic sometimes used to treat bacterial vaginosis, some physicians report a high success rate, even with women who fail to respond to metronidazole.

As with trichomonas vaginitis, if you are pregnant you will need to talk to your physician about being given a drug other than metronidazole to treat your bacterial vaginosis. And, also as with trichomonas vaginitis, bacterial vaginosis can complicate pregnancy. According to a 1992 article in *Clinical Infectious Diseases,* "Bacterial vaginosis has been widely assumed to be benign and asymptomatic cases often are not treated. However, recent data have linked the syndrome with acute pelvic inflammatory disease, premature rupture of the fetal membranes, and related complications of labor and delivery."

Lactobacillus acidophilus supplements may also help in the treatment of bacterial vaginosis. In their essay on the vaginal microflora of women, published in *Vulvovaginal Infections*, Roger L. Cook, Ph.D., Vincente Redondo-Lopez, M.D., and Jack D. Sobel, M.D., write that lactobacilli that are normally present in the vagina protect against the overgrowth of potentially harmful organisms. Research cited by Drs. Cook, Redondo-Lopez, and Sobel further emphasizes the importance of naturally occurring lactobacilli in the body and the possible (but unproven) helpfulness of *Lactobacillus acidophilus* supplements, especially in treating bacterial vaginosis. Drs. Cook, Redondo-Lopez, and Sobel write: "The pathogenesis [development] of bacterial vaginosis is thought to include the elimination or reduction of antibacterial activity expressed by indigenous vaginal lactobacilli. Lactobacilli were able to inhibit the in vitro growth of vaginosis-associated bacteria, including *Gardnerella, Mobiluncus,* peptostreptococci and *Bacteroides.*"

Recurrent Vaginal Infections

No matter which treatments are used, about 15 to 20 percent of women with vaginitis (less than 5 percent of the entire population) do not respond to the treatments available and are categorized as having difficult-to-treat vaginal infections. Women who have four or more confirmed infections during a one-year period are considered to have recurrent vaginitis.

Many women with CRC have persistent vaginal infections, so there is a big chance that the cause of their problems is the same one that allows them to have this problem in the first place: a weakened immune system that cannot control the Candida in their bodies. If this is the case, as the normal treatment for CRC progresses, the infections should go away along with the other CRC symptoms. However, if you have recurrent vaginal infections or problems, it is a good idea to examine the possibilities for recurrent vaginitis listed later in this chapter, just in case they apply to you. In order to rule out some of the possibilities you will need to talk to your doctor. After their CRC is under control, women who previously had vaginal infections should not have them at all..However, they may happen infrequently or during high-risk times, such as during pregnancy or if birth control pills or antibiotics are taken. If your infections continue to happen after your CRC is under control, be sure to go to your gynecologist for further advice and treatment.

Although a small percentage of women have always had problems with recurrent infections, the number of vaginal infections in general and women with recurrent infections has greatly increased during the 1980s and 1990s. Unfortunately, recurrent vaginitis in otherwise healthy women is poorly understood by the medical community. Despite a great deal of research that has been put into why vaginal infections recur after treatment, some questions have been answered, but many more have not. Recurrent infections also appear to be very individual. No one answer or discovery will apply to all women who suffer from recurrent vaginitis. But, as Dr. Sobel writes in *Vulvovaginal Infections*, women with recurrent Candidal vaginitis are different from women with infrequent vaginitis because they are incapable of tolerating certain amounts of Candida reintroduced or existing in their vagina.

When it comes to recurrent infections, there are many questions involved, and answering all of them will take time. Recent research appears to have answered one of the most important questions concerning recurrent infections, although additional studies will no doubt be done to confirm these findings. The question was whether or not new infections were simply relapses of old infections, or if they were actually caused by reinfection with a different Candida strain. This question is crucial because it affects the way physicians should treat recurrent infections. A prolonged treatment is more appropriate for an existing strain, and a short treatment regimen is effective for a newly acquired strain. A study, which concluded that recurrent infections are much more likely to be relapses of the original infecting strain than a new strain, was published in 1991 in *Diagnostic Microbiology and Infectious Diseases*. The authors used a recently developed epidemiological typing system to investigate the individual strains of *Candida albicans* in women with recurrent vaginitis. The study found that recurrent infections are often due to the relapse of the original infecting strain, not a new strain brought over from the rectum. This research supports the practice by most doctors to treat recurrent infections with prolonged treatment regimens in an effort to fully cure the patient.

Another important question that has recently been answered concerns drug resistance and whether or not it plays a part in recurrent episodes of Candidal vaginitis. This question is especially important because many women are treated for long periods of time with antifungal drugs. A 1993 article in *Genitourinary Medicine* reports that of the 250 different strains of *Candida albicans* isolated from forty-four women, none showed resistance to any of the antifungal agents tested. This study supports other studies that have found strains of *Candida albicans* in women with recurrent vaginitis that are not resistant to antifungal drugs. However, research has shown that some non-albicans species of Candida do show resistance to antifungal drugs commonly used to treat *Candida albicans* and other Candida species. Although they are not usually a big problem in regard to vaginal infections, other yeast species, such as *Saccharomyces cerevisiae*, are more resistant to common antifungal drugs.

Possible Reasons for Recurrent Vaginal Infections

Although what actually triggers an infection might be unknown, an infection is simply the result of a change in the ecology of the vagina. Since any number of factors can change the ecology of the vagina, there are numerous things that cause recurrent vaginal infections. If none of the reasons below seems to fit your individual case, don't be discouraged. As Dr. Sobel said in his book, unfortunately no underlying or predisposing factors can be identified in the majority of women with recurrent Candidal vaginal infections. When factors can be identified, however, they include these possibilities:

You may have an undiagnosed or mixed infection: If you haven't already had diagnostic tests performed for bacterial vaginosis and trichomonas vaginitis, these tests and other tests for sexually transmitted diseases should be performed to rule out the possibility of a mixed infection.

You may have diabetes: This is not a very strong possibility, since diabetes isn't often associated with CRC. In *A Woman's Guide to*

Yeast Infections, Dr. Baumslag and Dia Michels report of the thousands of non-CRC patients who have recurrent vaginal infections and have been tested for diabetes, the percentage who have tested even slightly diabetic is close to zero. You may wish to ask your physician, but for the majority of women a glucose tolerance test for diabetes is not necessary.

Use of a diaphragm and/or spermicidal creams or contraceptive jellies: Women who use diaphragms and/or spermicidal creams or jellies are at a higher risk for infections by non-albicans species of Candida. Diaphragms, spermicidal creams, and contraceptive jellies disrupt the normal microflora in the vagina, and this can make it easier for non-albicans species of Candida to thrive and cause problems. Another possible risk associated with using a diaphragm is it can become contaminated with yeast or bacteria and reinfect the user. If you think this is possible in your case, talk to your doctor about getting another diaphragm or soak your diaphragm in an antiseptic solution recommended by your doctor.

Your Candidal infections may be sexually transmitted: Sexual transmission is suspected to be responsible for a small amount of recurrent infections in women. In general, treating the sexual partner does not seem to stop recurrent Candidal infections, but if your partner has a discharge from his penis or abnormal swelling, he may need treatment. Approximately 20 percent of the male partners of women with recurrent Candidal vaginitis have asymptomatic penile colonization.

You may have an infection by a non-albicans species of Candida: Although the majority of Candida infections are caused by *Candida albicans,* infections by other species, such as *Candida tropicalis* and *Candida glabrata,* are increasing. Non-albicans species of Candida are not always destroyed by medications designed for *Candida albicans.*

Although the reasons for non-albicans infections are being investigated and nothing has been proven yet, two theories are possible. The first is that the drugs often used to treat vaginal infections are incapable of killing non-albicans species of Candida. This allows non-albicans species not only to survive, but possibly to thrive because their competition (*Candida albicans*) is gone. This theory is supported by research that has been conducted on commonly used antifungal drugs. The second reason is that although shorter courses of antifungal therapy kill *Candida albicans,* the shortened therapies allow less susceptible organisms to grow out of control. The result is a disrupted vaginal environment, which may be all non-albicans species of Candida need to grow and multiply.

So far, research has indicated that different strains of Candida are not necessarily more virulent than *Candida albicans*, but that the medications that kill *Candida albicans* do not always kill other Candida species. The recurrence rate for non-albicans species of Candida is also higher than the recurrence rate for *Candida albicans*. A 1992 article in the *Journal of Clinical Pharmacology* reports that the recurrence rate for *Candida tropicalis* is 33 percent, while the recurrence rate for *Candida albicans* after treatment is 16 percent.

You may have altered immunity: This possibility is very likely because many CRC patients have weak immune systems or immune systems that specifically cannot fight off Candida. Research suggests that women who suffer from repeated incidents of vaginitis, but who are otherwise healthy, have altered immunity. Constant or recurrent infections also weaken the body's ability to fight off infections. A study involving twenty-three women with recurrent vaginitis found that while their cells that digest invading microorganisms work correctly, peripheral blood lymphocytes have a delayed response to Candida. Another study showed the same results, with the peripheral blood lymphocytes having "reduced or absent proliferative responses to Candida antigens." Given this, it makes sense to boost immune system defenses through vitamins and a low-sugar diet while continuing antifungal treatment.

Avoiding Recurrent Vaginal Infections

The suggestions on how to prevent vaginal infections in general also apply to preventing recurrent infections. However, with recurrent infections, there is a greater need to anticipate infections and treat them prophylactically. If your infections fall into a predictable pattern, anticipate and treat them with nonprescription vaginal creams and suppositories, or with medications prescribed by your physician. Many women report that they are more likely to develop an infection between ovulation and the onset of their menses. If that is true for you, take actions to prevent an infection from occurring. Taking antibiotics can also trigger a vaginal infection, so be sure to take acidophilus supplements before, during, and after you take the antibiotics.

If you have persistent problems with vaginal infections, do not overly depend on nonprescription products if you really need stronger medications. By using smaller amounts of more effective medications, you may actually be saving yourself money. Ask your gynecologist for advice on how to develop a suppressive maintenance regimen for preventing infections. Several studies on women with recurrent vaginitis have shown that once they have gone into full remission, 50 percent of women relapse after three months and 75 percent after six months. In his 1990 article published in the

Journal of the American Academy of Dermatology, Dr. Sobel said that maintenance therapy can be topical or oral, and can be given daily or less frequently. He also said that the maintenance regimens that have been the most successful are those with a daily or weekly administration of an antifungal agent. Dr. Sobel reports that the best suppression maintenance has been attained with daily low-dose oral ketoconazole therapy, although similar results can also be achieved with the newer triazole drugs. Dr. Sobel describes the maintenance regimens as not truly curative, but actually effective suppressive agents. By suppressing the problem, maintenance regimens allow women to lead normal lives and sometimes allow the body to heal itself through its natural defense mechanisms.

A maintenance regimen doesn't have to be expensive or complicated, and can be administered in the form of suppositories or oral tablets. According to Dr. Sobel, three examples of successful maintenance regimens are 100mg of ketoconazole daily, 500mg clotrimazole suppositories once a week, and 100mg orally of fluconazole once a week.

Tips for Preventing Vaginal Infections

It is a good idea to follow these suggestions as much as possible, not just when you believe you may have a vaginal infection. In addition to the following recommendations, taking acidophilus supplements regularly will not only help you feel better, it will also help protect you from vaginal infections. Here are some additional suggestions:

- Eat a balanced and nutritious diet to help your body resist infection.
- Reduce the amount of sugar in your diet. Sugar promotes yeast growth, and high levels of sugar can change the normal pH level of your vagina.
- Avoid using other people's towels or personal items.
- Use mild and unscented bath soap and laundry detergent.
- Add a small amount of bleach to your laundry to help kill Candida on your underwear.
- Use tampons instead of pads during your period. Not only do pads shut off air flow to the vagina, they also retain moisture—two things that encourage Candida growth. However, avoid superabsorbent tampons and scented or deodorant tampons and be sure to change your tampons every several hours.
- Avoid using spermicides, which can be irritating or trigger vaginitis. If you wish to use a spermicide, put it in the reservoir tip of your partner's latex condom.

- Wipe your anal area from front to back to decrease the chance that bacteria from the anus will enter the vaginal area.
- Avoid douching unless recommended by your doctor. Douching can push harmful organisms farther into your reproductive system.
- Wear clean all-cotton underwear, which allows for maximum air circulation.
- Avoid pantyhose and nylon underwear which can help bacteria grow by retaining moisture and heat.
- Avoid pants that are tight in the crotch and thighs. Keep your vaginal area as ventilated as possible. This includes not wearing several layers of clothing and sleeping naked or without panties under your nightgown.
- Keep the vagina clean and dry, and wash your vulva and anus regularly. Instead of using soaps, which can be drying, try using pure and unscented mineral oil, which does not dry out skin, or just wash with water. Avoid using talcum powder, bubble bath, bath oil, and feminine hygiene sprays because they can be irritating and even harmful.

If your vagina or any part of your genital area is sore, or if you or your partner have a genital infection, don't attempt sexual intercourse. If you do have intercourse, use an unlubricated and unribbed condom to prevent transmitting an infection. If lubrication is needed during intercourse, use mineral oil or a sterile, water-soluble jelly. Do not use Vaseline, which can cause small holes to form in the rubber of the condom, or baby oil, because it contains potentially irritating additives.

INFORMATION AND ADVICE

—14—

Coping and Living with CRC

Everything can be taken from a man but one thing: the last of the human freedoms—to choose one's attitude in any given set of circumstances, to choose one's own way.
—Viktor Frankl in *Man's Search for Meaning*

Truly coping and living with CRC involves changing the way you structure and live your life. As we all know, CRC is not a minor illness that requires just a few days of rest and some offhand medical care. Because of its complexity, CRC can last anywhere from a few months to several years and can be both confusing and discouraging. Recovery from CRC involves freeing yourself from ideas you have been conditioned to believe, such as the following:

- We, as patients, can eat whatever we want without consequences.
- As patients, we should be docile and not ask for explanations or bother busy physicians with questions.
- Ill health is a simple imbalance that can be corrected with pills, surgery, and other quick-fix methods.

No one says living with CRC is easy, but many patients who have recovered emphasize that their lives are healthier, more rewarding, and more satisfying. In *Minding the Body, Mending the Mind* Joan Borysenko, Ph.D., tells the story of former Olympic medalist, skier Jimmy Huega, whose exhilarating career ended when he developed multiple sclerosis (MS). She writes:

187

After sinking into a debilitating depression, he realized that he had a choice. He could be a healthy person with MS or an unhealthy person with MS. He began a program of regular physical exercise (which varies with his daily energy level and the course of his MS), proper nutrition, and meditation. His view of himself is as a superiorly healthy person who also has MS. What is your view of yourself? Is inner peace completely dependent on bodily condition?

Jimmy Huega's story demonstrates that when it comes to living and coping with a chronic illness, many choices are available. By now we all know there are no quick cures for CRC, and the treatment is long and even difficult. The choices are yours:

- You can decide not to follow the recommended treatments and live with whatever level of health you had before being diagnosed with CRC. Often patients delay treatment because eating unhealthy meals and neglecting themselves suit the fast-paced life they lead.

- You can take antifungal medicine, all the recommended supplements, sometimes follow the Candida control diet, and maintain a minimal level of health.

- Or, like Jimmy Huega, you can be a healthy person who also happens to have an illness. But doing so means remembering that to half follow the treatment is to fully cheat yourself, and everyone around you, out of your best chances for a total recovery.

The whole treatment, all the little-yet-necessary bits and pieces, the big medications, and the little remedies, is what gets and keeps sick people well. Getting to the final point, the point of recovery, involves sticking with all the treatments outlined in this book and truly being motivated to get and stay well. The Candida control diet is, of course, often the hardest and longest therapy to follow, especially since as adults we are all accustomed to eating whatever we want whenever we want.

Coping and living with CRC, for a short or long period of time, are challenges many physicians who treat CRC assume will be taken care of by each patient in his or her own fashion. As Kathy Charmaz writes in *Good Days, Bad Days: The Self in Chronic Illness and Time*, "As a logical consequence of fragmentation within the medical care system, people commonly handle illnesses in individualistic, idiosyncratic ways, frequently in isolation and with little information."

Physicians feel more comfortable focusing on physiological rather than psychological problems and assume patients will know how and where to seek out the assistance they need. Because CRC is different from other medical conditions, however, patients sometimes have trouble contending and living with the difficulties CRC can cause in their lives. This is both understandable and normal given that any chronic illness has the ability to turn a structured, ordinary life upside down.

Coping and living with CRC aren't easy but, just as all other aspects of recovery are up to the patient, handling the psychological impact of CRC is also each patient's responsibility. Given advice and skills, however, adjusting to CRC doesn't have to be painful or even difficult.

How a Chronic Illness Changes Your Life

Because CRC incapacitates some people but is not debilitating for others, the process of living with CRC varies from patient to patient. In fact, if you have already been living with CRC from anywhere from months to years, you have probably already changed your life in small and big ways because of your health problems. In *Good Days, Bad Days: The Self in Chronic Illness and Time*, Charmaz explores what people learn and how their lives change when they experience a chronic illness. Charmaz's interest in chronic illness began when she worked as an occupational therapist with people who had physical disabilities. She is a faculty member at Sonoma State University in California.

After interviewing close to one hundred people and having informal discussions with many more, Charmaz summarizes the ways in which people's lives change when they have to live with a chronic illness. She describes living with a chronic illness as a process that involves merging the illness with strategies that keep the illness contained and keep independence from being lost. Living with a chronic illness changes your life in three important ways:

- The *context* of your life changes, which means the actual way and manner in which you live your life change to adapt to your illness. Often people develop creative strategies as a way to complete the tasks they never had problems completing before they became ill.

- Your life is *remade* and reorganized so control and independence are not sacrificed.

- A necessary part of living with a chronic illness is to make *trade-offs* that make a more complicated life manageable and allow people to get through the day. Often these trade-offs are made to simplify life, to help with a reordering of time and the making of a schedule, and to accommodate the necessary balancing and pacing of activities.

Depending on whether their CRC is a chronic problem or a nagging inconvenience, patients frequently find that getting through the day means developing strategies to compensate for their reduced capacity for work and delicate health. In fact, living with a chronic illness is in itself a strategy, with all plans and activities directed toward the immediate task of getting through each day without overexerting yourself. Although living your life day by day is important, your primary goal has to be regaining your health. While you may be able to get by at work or take care of the children by using clever strategies and plans, it is extremely important that you remember not to strain your health. Keep in mind, your daily goal is to prevent your health from getting worse, while your long-term goal is to regain your health.

Changing the Context of Your Life

Living with a chronic illness means changing the fabric and shape of your life. Change is inevitable. It is, in fact, the only constant in life. Living with an illness simply means working around more variables and changes than you had before your illness. When describing how people smoothly adapt to the illness in their life, sometimes without even noticing, Charmaz writes:

> As a result, ill people become innovators in handling their illnesses, inventors of their lives, and creators of ways of coping. Not surprisingly, some of their inventions remain taken for granted and unnoted. Furthermore, they do not think of other possibilities or realize when they might have choices. Rather, their inventions and adaptations flow together in what eventually feels natural.

Because we are accustomed to change, it is only natural for us not to notice all the rapidly occurring changes in our lives. When you are ill everything is different: your needs, your relationships with the people around you, and most importantly, your feelings about yourself become less secure. Often the inability to take care of routine tasks is seen by patients as a representation of their limitations and their changed feelings toward their own self-worth. These feelings are normal; they are simply the result of a restructuring of your life.

Re-creating Your Life

Often the problems associated with chronic illness can be managed by focusing on and organizing what needs to be accomplished. As

Charmaz writes, "The problems with which ill people struggle are existential; their solutions are often organizational."

Most people find that living with CRC means developing strategies and plans, and then changing them as the days or months go on. Without these strategies and plans, their independence is threatened. These strategies may include how to conceal your illness from everyone other than your immediate family, how to accomplish small tasks, or even how to juggle your finances so you can afford the medications you need. Planning is another crucial element. For example, patients who are allergic to chemicals and personal-scent products may have to go to the grocery store in the very early morning so as to avoid contact with other people. Or, they may not be able to go to the grocery store at all and have to rely on someone else to do the shopping and other chores. Making complex plans helps patients feel they have retained control over their lives.

One facet of reorganizing your life includes making reasonable decisions about your life. Too often dreams and hopes have to be delayed until health can be regained. "Learning effective organization depends upon fitting activities between hopes and plans," writes Charmaz. "This often means scaling down hopes and former expectations of self and planning around disability."

Many women who become ill find they can no longer work outside the home and still manage to take care of all the household and child-rearing duties. Because of this, the responsibility for organizing household tasks is taken over by other members of the family. For example, if a woman is ill, her husband takes on more household chores, or if a man is sick, his wife adds some of his chores to her own. Children also pitch in and add new tasks to their household routines. Another common routine is for the ill person to continue to make decisions and simply delegate them to other members of the family. This shifting of responsibilities frequently enables the ill person to continue to work outside the home and bring in necessary income.

Making Trade-Offs: A Key to Survival
A necessary part of reordering your life has to do with making trade-offs. That is, deciding not only what can and cannot be done, but also what tasks or goals are most important and which can be omitted. This is done by simplifying life, by restructuring time and making schedules, and by balancing activities and pacing yourself so as not to strain your health.

Simplifying your life means making your life easier. This is done by cutting out everything that isn't absolutely necessary in order to reduce work and stress. There is still a price to pay, however, because the things you decide to give up wouldn't have been part of your life in the first place if they weren't meaningful in some way. While making trade-offs can be hard, it is a necessary part of restructuring your life. "Changes, compromises, and sacrifices permit ill people to carry on a life, albeit a simplified one. That's the trade-off," explains Charmaz. Reducing your life to the essentials means paying for services you once did yourself or consolidating many tasks into fewer tasks. Some examples are having a cleaning service clean your house or having a relative or friend buy food for you. Relaxing pursuits, such as shopping, reading, and gardening, don't have to be eliminated from a busy schedule, only reduced or simplified.

Restructuring, planning, and scheduling your life are further steps toward successfully living with a chronic illness. Creating a structured and orderly routine where one didn't exist before is a trade-off that helps get you through the day. For example, staying up late at night, skipping meals, and eating junk food are behaviors that once would not have negatively affected your health, but now they do. Rearranging your life to ensure you get the sleep and food you need might be tedious, but it will help you in the long run. Being able to complete the tasks that are part of the schedule will also help build your self-confidence.

Pacing your activities so as not to exhaust yourself is another organizational talent that prevents shaky health from worsening. Often people who develop CRC have led very hectic lives, and learning to slow down and reduce your responsibilities can be a formidable task. Often pacing has to be combined with juggling of activities so that neither the activities nor your health will be sacrificed.

Coping with CRC

Coping is managing the demands upon us. Because we all come from different backgrounds, our coping skills vary from person to person. We learn how to cope or how not to cope from watching our parents and family and how they handle the daily stresses in their lives. Our culture, our level of education, even the geographical area we live in all influence how we control and order our lives. Our physiology also contributes to our reactions to stress. As Dr. Sehnert points out in his international best-seller *How to Be Your Own Doctor (Sometimes)*, "Tall, lanky ectomorphic types tend to respond to pressure with their stomachs, and end up with ulcers. The heavily muscled mesomorph body type tends to take his troubles to heart—he's coronary-prone. Stress seems to search out the flaw in the balloon, wherever it may be."

Research indicates that coping effectively with an illness helps patients stay healthy. In a study of cancer patients and coping skills conducted at the University of California at Los Angeles (UCLA), researchers found that patients who were able to learn effective coping skills were healthier several years later than patients who were not as proficient at adapting and coping with their cancer. This study on coping was the first ever to evaluate coping combined with the onset of illness. The findings indicate something that has long been suspected: cognitive and behavioral changes have an incredible impact on the outcome of an illness or disease.

By the time we are adults, we have all been exposed to stress of one form or another, from our jobs, families, friendships, relationships, and numerous other sources. But often men and women who never had problems coping with life's daily stresses find themselves overwhelmed by CRC. While the psychological effects of any illness are profound, CRC seems to be not only different, but also to have a unique impact.

The Psychological Effects of CRC
Simply put, the psychological effects of CRC on the patient come from two sources: the medical condition itself and the inability of some people around the patient to understand and cope with the medical condition categories. Between these two forces it isn't surprising that many patients have difficulty overcoming the obstacles CRC creates in their lives.

As discussed previously, CRC does not fit neatly into recognizable and predictable symptoms or categories and causes mental and psychological symptoms as well as physical ones. The psychological symptoms are very profound and include depression, fatigue, feelings of spaciness, a sense of unrealness, irritability, agitation, anxiety, and nervousness. As if these psychological symptoms weren't enough, most CRC patients also have to contend with an initial lack of understanding and help from both the medical community and their family and friends.

Most illnesses are recognized and heavily studied by the medical community and at least partially understood by the general public. Most people are even vaguely familiar with fairly recent illnesses such as Chronic Fatigue Syndrome (CFS) and Lyme disease. Unfortunately, since so few people are aware of CRC, it tends to isolate the sufferers and makes coping with CRC unlike living with any other medical condition.

There are several additional reasons why living with CRC is unlike living with other medical conditions. Simply put, these reasons specifically concern how this problem differs from our concept of illness and the fact that CRC still hasn't been accepted by mainstream medicine. The reasons are spelled out here:

- *The nature of CRC.* We are accustomed to diseases that have either physical or mental symptoms. CRC causes both types of symptoms, which makes it difficult to understand and sometimes hard to explain to the people in your life. Candida-related symptoms are also very diverse, which also causes confusion. Symptoms can not only vary from person to person, but they can also vary from time to time for a single patient.

- *CRC tends to isolate patients from their loved ones and from society.* The difficulty people have understanding CRC is partially responsible for the fact that people both in the medical community and outside it are unfamiliar with this complex illness. Because many people are unaware of CRC, and because the physical and mental symptoms patients experience can be hard to understand, they may tend to disbelieve patients or hint that they are exaggerating their problems. This can lead to withdrawal from people and society.

- *CRC tends to isolate patients from mainstream medicine.* The typical patient who has just been diagnosed with CRC has most likely suffered incapacitating symptoms for many years. The response from the medical community has been a diagnosis of "it's all in your head," which conveniently ends the attending physician's responsibility. This constant denial of the patient's feelings and problems often leads to distrust, discontent, and eventually isolation from mainstream medicine.

- *Finding a physician can be difficult.* Because CRC still hasn't been accepted by mainstream medicine, patients also often find it difficult to find a physician who is both knowledgeable about CRC and sympathetic to what they are going through. The majority of physicians are unaware of the tremendous power and influence they have on their patients' lives and actions.

These reasons have one unifying factor: unless the patient has a sympathetic physician and an understanding family, the responsibility for coping with, understanding, and treating the illness rests solely on the patient's shoulders. Given the profound psychological stress CRC puts on patients, it is no wonder many have problems coping with the changes CRC creates in their lives.

These stresses wear down the psychological defenses of all patients, from the most psychologically strong to the most psychologically strained. They also have a profound psychological effect on the medical community's acceptance of CRC, on the patient and his or her progress, and on the patient's family and friends. Given these difficulties and the sweeping lifestyle changes necessary to improve their health, it isn't surprising many patients feel discouraged and may have problems coping with their CRC.

Three Strategies for Effectively Coping with CRC

To successfully cope with CRC you need three tools: information, motivation, and support. Without these three things there is a greater chance of failure, and repeated failures can damage your self-confidence and keep you from improving.

All three tools are linked together and enhance each other. Information, of course, means educating yourself about your health problems through finding and reading books and articles. Physicians, fellow patients, and support groups are also great sources for advice on medications and different methods of treatment. By gathering information and learning as much as you can about CRC, you will know what to expect in the future and gain confidence in yourself and your ability to treat not only your present medical problems, but new ones should they come along. Seeking out information is the first step toward taking control of your life and health and will help give you the motivation you need to continue to properly take care of yourself. Once motivated to control your health you can successfully seek out the support you need.

Information: An Important First Step
Gathering information is your first step toward being in charge of your health. Remember the old saying that states the best defense against an opponent is a good offense? By learning as much as you can about CRC, you are moving toward taking control of both your health and your life. In a study of cancer patients, the most well-adjusted patients took an active role in their health by talking more to their physicians and by finding out as much information as they could about their illness. Patients who took a more passive or resigned role tended to be anxious and depressed. Try to inform yourself by reading as many books and articles as you can and by talking to as many people in your area who have CRC as possible. Focus your attention on what will help you the most: if you experience environmental symptoms, buy books on environmental illness. If food allergies or digestive problems are your biggest difficulty, then find articles or books on these topics.

If you can't find a support group or CRC contact person in your area, try putting a personal ad in the newspaper or try contacting local alternative-medicine physicians or chiropractors to see if they know of any CRC patients or even support groups in the area. For many people health food stores provide more than necessary food and medical items; they also provide information and advice. Because most health food stores are small, service tends to be more personal, and employees and regular customers are more likely to develop personal relationships. Visit and speak to the employees (or even the customers) about what over-the-counter treatments seem to be especially helpful for CRC patients. Health food store personnel may also be able to refer you to local doctors who treat CRC and may be able to volunteer recent information on CRC medicines or products.

You may also want to ask your local health food store if you can try to contact other CRC patients by posting a notice on its bulletin board, or if the employees can keep your name and address behind the counter in case any other CRC patients express a similar need for telephone or personal contact.

Taking control of your CRC is your first big step in the right direction. When you know a great deal about CRC you will understand what needs to be done and the changes you will need to make in your life. The point is for you to take control of both your illness and your life and help yourself. Once you have recognized what you need to do and have confidence in your ability to handle the new challenges in your life, you will know what to expect and you will have the motivation you need to start or continue treatment.

Motivation: The Force that Keeps Us All Going

Why do some people have trouble complying with the treatment necessary for CRC? There are several reasons patients fail to begin treatment, or begin treatment but stop midway. First of all, there is limited access to treatment. Physicians who treat CRC and the necessary products available at health food stores can sometimes be difficult to find. Another common problem is the inability to afford treatment. Patients without health insurance or whose health insurance refuses to cover physicians who practice alternative medicine may find they will have trouble affording their CRC treatment. A third reason is the adverse physical and mental effects of treatment. One example is the die-off process that is common during the initial stages of treatment. During die-off, which is a normal reaction to treatments, patients often experience a general worsening of all symptoms, and the process can be extremely difficult to go through.

Effectively coping and living with CRC mean being prepared to make major lifestyle changes and restrictions. People preparing themselves to make lifestyle changes are more likely to make gradual rather than immediate and full progress. Keep in mind that small changes are in some ways as important as big changes. Handling your CRC is not an all-or-nothing situation. The goal doesn't have to be to change your entire life overnight, but just to *change*. Any and all change is progress in the right direction.

Lapses, relapses, and struggling are natural and necessary parts of change. A lapse is a slight slip backward while a relapse is a return to a previous state. Understanding why you faltered will help prevent further lapses. Don't see lapses as failures, but rather as ways to learn new coping skills and as an opportunities to reexamine your situation.

Before you make big changes you have to know what it is about your life you want to change and you have to be ready to change. No one—not your physician, not your friends, not even your family—can motivate you unless you are ready and willing to change. Once you know what you want, you can set goals and make yourself stick to them. Another good idea is to periodically evaluate your health. It is crucial to remember that only you can accept responsibility for your recovery. Although physicians, friends, and family can and should help, only you can make the necessary lifestyle changes you need to survive.

Support: The Glue that Keeps Everything Together

Talk to people and actively seek support. Don't try to deal with this yourself: it is important to fully involve your friends and family. Too many times patients pretend nothing is wrong or act as if they can handle CRC by themselves. Many believe that to tell others about their CRC would be a sign of weakness. Having such an attitude, however, will only alienate people who care about you and may also delay your recovery. A professional counselor is a very good idea because friends and family can become tired and lose patience with lengthy discussions of your health problems. Ministers, psychiatrists, doctors, or personnel at a mental health clinic are all trained to be good listeners.

Your family will need time to adjust and to fully understand what you are going through. Mark Fowler and Gloria Axelrod make an important contribution on this topic in *Candida* by Dr. De Schepper. They urge CRC patients to be tolerant with friends and family: "The first thing to realize is that it's very difficult for them to understand and appreciate a disease they've never had, can't see, and [have] never even heard of!" Your friends and family want to help you, but keep in mind that just as your CRC is an added complication in your life, it is also another snarl in their lives. This doesn't mean you shouldn't include them, it just means they may need time and help in accepting the new changes in your life.

Support is crucial to your recovery. Studies show that patients with supportive families or a network of supportive friends have less depression and better recovery rates. Both emotional support and helpful actions such as giving rides to the doctor's office, running errands, and helping patients prepare meals are extremely important.

Living with CRC

Just as coping with CRC is often a new experience, living with CRC can be a big adjustment because for most patients the lifestyle changes involved are both required and permanent. In general, living with this condition means you have to take better care of yourself.

As we all race toward our goals, too often we forget to take care of ourselves, and nothing could be more essential for recovery than taking care of both your mind and body. Set up a regular program for meals, breaks, exercise, relaxation, fun, and rest. Once you set up a regular schedule and include your family and friends in it, straying from the schedule will be difficult. Here are eleven additional suggestions to keep in mind:

- Self-respect is a must. You need to have faith in your own ability to solve problems. Once you have started successfully coping with your CRC, your self-respect will increase.

- Anxiety is a perfectly normal emotion, but it isn't very productive. The best way for you to handle anxiety is to stop it early on. When you start to feel anxious, first determine and then correct whatever is causing your anxiety. In his landmark book *Stress Without Distress*, Hans Selye, M.D., cautions people to make sure the stresses in their lives are really worth the trouble they cause. As Dr. Sehnert writes in *Stress/Unstress*, "Avoid hurry, flurry, worry. These far too common lifestyles alter your patterns of eating, sleeping, working and recreation. They are learned habits and can be unlearned." He continues, writing that stress, like anxiety, should be directly confronted. Set aside time to think and plan about the events, places, or people who regularly cause you stress and anxiety.

- Regular exercise is crucial to regaining your health. Choose whatever type of exercise best suits your physical condition, fitness level, and schedule, whether it's walking, jogging, hiking, biking, aerobics, calisthenics, or any other activity or sport.

- Relaxation is a key to survival for everyone, both healthy and ill. Many people exercise to relax, or listen to music. Many others watch TV, rent a movie, write a letter, make a phone call, do a little bit of recreational shopping, or even just get out of the house. Because it is impossible to be both relaxed and anxious at the same time, relaxation should be an important part of each day.

- Identify and confront your fears by seeking information. Fear is simply apprehension of the unknown, so learning more about an uncertain event or future occurrence will lessen your fear. The pressure to make decisions can also cause anxiety. Just as stress doesn't come from outside or around us, but rather from inside each one of us, the solution for every problem is also inside us.

- Write out your fears, hopes, worries, dreams, achievements, anxieties, and all other thoughts every day in a journal or diary. Often keeping a journal and expressing yourself in a personal and private manner will help you move beyond your daily crisises and at the same time help you recognize patterns you didn't know existed. For example, you might realize that a certain person or daily event causes you undue stress and be able to eliminate or mitigate that stress in the future.

- Don't hesitate or be afraid to compromise when it seems the best solution. As Dr. Sehnert writes, "In a stressful situation you can either fight, back off, or compromise. Seldom is the ideal situation available."

- Try to rethink the situation and see it from a different perspective. Many people recovering from CRC look back at the adjustments they had to make in their lives, and although they still remember the changes as being difficult and even painful to make, they are now able to view their present habits as beneficial and their health as better than it has ever been.

- Appreciate what you have. Too often we look forward or beyond ourselves to what we cannot have or will never get and forget the good things in our lives, such as good jobs, loving family relationships, and caring friends. Appreciate what you have and take the time to talk to and listen to your loved ones.

- Take action to change or control what you can. Resisting the inevitable is pointless, but every situation contains variables that you can use to control your circumstances to some degree. Even little actions and goals move us forward and closer to improved health.

- Because emotions, both positive and negative, greatly affect our health, it is important to be as positive and hopeful as possible. In *Head First: The Biology of Hope and the Healing Power of the Human Spirit*, Norman Cousins emphasizes the need for improved patient involvement in the struggle with disease. He also said, "Patients tend to move along the path of their expectations, whether on the upside or on the downside."

Cousins, a former professor of medicine at UCLA, spent years studying the effects of emotions on health. He wrote, "A strong will to live, along with the other positive emotions—faith, love, purpose, determination, humor—are biochemical realities that can affect the environment of medical care. The positive emotions are no less a physiological factor on the upside than are the negative emotions on the downside." In his book, Cousins repeatedly emphasizes the beneficial effects positive emotions play in helping patients overcome their diseases. Although a cheerful demeanor and a hopeful outlook do not ensure a complete reversal of a disease, they do greatly help patients overcome their health problems. At the very least, he notes, "They (positive attitudes) can create an environment conducive to medical care and can enable both patient and physician to get the most out of whatever may be possible."

When Others Have Trouble Understanding

Having to handle other people's negative reactions to your health problem is, unfortunately, often a difficult and unavoidable part of having an illness. Because CRC can be difficult to understand and explain, people may seem to criticize or reprimand you for having a medical condition you can't help having and are doing your best to overcome. Often when people don't understand a medical condition or problem, they emotionally or physically draw away from the patient.

Although facing and communicating with potentially negative people can be difficult, the experience can be mentally stimulating and rewarding. As Joan Borysenko, Ph.D., author of *Minding the Body, Mending the Minds* writes: "You cannot control the external circumstances of your life, but you can control your reactions to them." She suggests that when faced with trying circumstances try turning the problem around: instead of seeing it as a threat, see it as a challenge. She explains, "In this way you acknowledge and nourish your own inner strength, even as you face doubt and uncertainty. Adversity is the crucible in which the spirit is forged."

Alan J. Levy, an associate professor of social work at Loyola

University in Chicago, stresses the need for patients to successfully cope with the stigma associated with having a chronic illness. Levy suggests five different approaches to what he calls "stigma management." Before you try them, however, make sure you are confident, emotionally ready to accept negative consequences (should they occur), and have a strong sense of self-assurance.

The first method Levy recommends is to *explore disclosure*. This involves identifying the circumstances in which you feel the most comfortable talking about your CRC and how illness affects your social interaction. Another approach is to *get support by association*, which means surrounding yourself with people who have situations similar to your own. Having people around you who can relate to your own experiences and feelings will reinforce your identity and relieve feelings of loneliness and separation.

A third way to lessen negative reactions to your illness is to *change the frame of reference*. By presenting your situation in a positive frame of reference, people will more easily understand it, and there is less chance of miscommunication. There are several ways to do this, but the easiest includes using examples and language people can understand and identify with.

Another strategy that helps people overcome their negative feelings toward your illness is to *evoke compassion* by emphasizing something you and they have in common, for example, relatives, friends, similar interests, jobs in related fields, or anything else you can think of at the time. Emphasizing whatever common ground you share will make your experiences and needs more important to them and will give you both other foundations upon which to build a relationship.

The final approach is to *directly confront* or challenge people who are giving you a difficult time. If someone is making you feel uncomfortable or upsetting you, remember that he may just be confused or uneasy. If someone is giving you a hard time, find a time when he or she will be alone and ask if he has questions about your health problems. Although one crucial goal is to try to get people to accept you and your CRC, another equally important goal is to improve your self-esteem and to empower yourself.

Although negative reactions to CRC are unavoidable, if people learn more about the situation and realize you need their support and compassion, they may make an effort to better help and understand your situation.

Living with a chronic illness means redefining yourself and your life. Unlike many chronically ill patients, CRC patients have something to look forward to: an end to their illness. It is because you have a chance at recovery that it is so important to strictly follow the Candida control diet and all the other therapies. While changing your life may be difficult, the opportunity to change is a chance many chronically ill patients, such as those who have cancer, AIDS, and countless other diseases, do not have. Living with an illness can be a difficult process, but if you take care of yourself it doesn't have to be a life sentence.

—15—

When to Use Antibiotics and Alternatives to Antibiotics

> *Whenever a new discovery is reported to the scientific world, they say first, "It is probably not true." Thereafter, when the truth of the new proposition has been demonstrated beyond question, they say, "Yes, it may be true, but it is not important." Finally, when sufficient time has elapsed to fully evidence its importance, they say, "Yes, surely it is important, but it is no longer new."*
>
> —Michel de Montaigne

All of the doctors who treat CRC agree that antibiotics are one of the most important factors, perhaps the most important, that contribute to CRC. Given this serious conclusion, it seems a good idea to avoid antibiotics whenever possible, and it is crucial that people who have CRC or who have recovered avoid antibiotics unless absolutely necessary.

So if we can't use antibiotics, what can we do? The answer is both simple and revolutionary. Many alternatives to antibiotics are available. Of course, they involve more effort than popping pills, but given the importance of good health, alternatives are more than worth simple consideration: they are worth extra effort.

Why Are Antibiotics Standard Medical Treatment?

The heavy use of antibiotics is simply a symptom of the way health is viewed and medicine practiced today. This is unfortunate because for so many CRC patients, the overuse of antibiotics contributed to or caused their CRC. And because of their resulting sensitivity to antibiotics, CRC patients must be extremely careful when taking antibiotics because to do so can aggravate current symptoms, cause additional symptoms, or cause a recovered patient to redevelop CRC. The need for experienced advice concerning CRC patients' use of antibiotics is another reason to pick a physician familiar with Candida. If a situation that involves antibiotics ever surfaces, she can help advise you on the best course of action for your unique condition.

Unfortunately, the way medicine is practiced in the twentieth century could accurately be described in terms of warfare instead of in terms of repair. Our contemporary approach to medicine began when the germ theory of disease became dominant, and the "kill it" attitude replaced the "work with the body" philosophy. These new attitudes gave medicine a new power, a new role, and allowed medicine to place itself and its theories before the individual's role in her own health. According to medicine today, the only responsibilities each individual has in her own health are to go to the doctor when sick and take the prescribed medications (a pill for every ill). Underlying causes of disease are seldom mentioned by the doctor to the patient. Preventative medicine is rarely practiced.

In an effort to treat illness, mainstream medicine attacks the body instead of working with it to heal and prevent disease. The fault for our many illnesses and diseases lies not with the microbial world but with our society, which has taken and continues to take the wrong approach to illness and disease. In *Alternative Medicine: The Definitive Guide*, by the Burton Goldberg Group, the authors describe modern medicine and in doing so also explain why the theories of modern medicine continue to fail us:

> Disease is considered an invasion by an enemy and treatment is aimed at developing 'magic bullets' in the forms of drugs and vaccines to eliminate the enemy. We have seen, for example, a failed 'war on cancer,' a proliferation of antibiotics, and a growing number of surgical procedures, cell-killing radiation treatments, and chemical medications (such as chemotherapy), all of which do harm to the body, in one form or another, in their attempts to restore health.

The consequences of the prevailing attitudes are simple: other, more common sense approaches have been overlooked or even squelched by "orthodox" medicine. According to the Burton Goldberg Group: "Lost in this approach is the concept of repairing the imbalances that allow the illnesses to occur in the first place.

Medical science has become one-sided in focus, increasingly losing sight of the whole person in its attempt to treat the body's individual parts."

Why are these attitudes toward health and healing important? Because they influence or determine the choices we all have when it comes to taking care of illnesses that are frequently treated with antibiotics.

Michael A. Schmidt, M.D., Lendon H. Smith, M.D., and Keith W. Sehnert, M.D., authors of *Beyond Antibiotics*, present more than information about antibiotics and alternatives to antibiotics: they offer common sense information about the various causes of and solutions to illness. They present four options to treating illness:

- To use antibiotics alone.
- To use antibiotics along with addressing the dietary, psychological, social, nutritional, lifestyle, and environmental contributors to illness.
- To avoid the use of antibiotics by addressing the contributors to illness noted above.
- To simply avoid becoming sick.

The first choice is both the most frequently chosen and the worst choice for three reasons. Simply using antibiotics alone neither confronts the underlying reasons for illness nor addresses the side effects of antibiotic use nor the effects infection can have on the body, such as nutrient and vitamin loss. Given the circumstances of the illness and the appropriateness of antibiotics for the situation, the second choice is a good option. The third option is equally viable, given that antibiotics can be avoided through nutritional or alternative treatments. The final option, avoiding illness altogether, is the best alternative and not as unattainable as popular opinion would have you believe. One example is to avoid foods known to cause food allergies. Another excellent example is the patient who has for the most part recovered from CRC and continues to follow the Candida control diet and the other lifestyle changes that enabled him or her to recover in the first place. Although this may seem like just common sense, the secret to good health is hardly a mystery. It is rather a logical conclusion given the role nutrition, diet, stress, proper rest, and other factors play in determining not only our daily well-being, but also our long-term health.

The importance of taking the responsibility for your own health into your own hands cannot be emphasized strongly enough. In chapter 16, when asked what they have learned from their experiences with CRC and what advice they would give someone with

CRC, patient after patient stressed the importance of relying on their own knowledge and skills instead of those of physicians. In his many books, Dr. Sehnert developed the concept of the activated patient, which describes the role and responsibilities each patient has in her own health care.

The three parts of the activated patient concept follow:

- People don't need a formal medical education to be trusted to take excellent care of their own health.
- Knowledge about health should not be a protected secret available only to health professionals, but rather should be shared with everyone, including patients.
- Given accurate information, ordinary people can treat a variety of common health problems earlier, cheaper, and in some cases more effectively than health professionals.

An acronym that describes activated patients is ABLE. To become an activated patient, you must do the following:

Accept more individual responsibility for your own and your family's care.

Become a wiser buyer and intelligent user of health-care services, medications, and nutritional options.

Learn how to observe and identify the meaning of different symptoms and, through experience and proper guidance, develop self-confidence in improving personal health.

Educate others about health attitudes, health promotion, stress management, self-care, exercise, and the environment so as to be a positive influence on health in general.

When illness does occur, it is important that both you and your physician are sure to consider two issues regarding the nature of the illness: whether or not the problem is a result of a bacterial infection (this requires that a culture be done), and if bacteria is present, what kind of bacteria it is.

Other questions you and your doctor should consider when trying to decide whether or not to use an antibiotic include the following:

- Which antibiotic will be most effective against the particular bacterium?
- If an antibiotic is necessary, is it best to take it immediately?
- What are the consequences, if any, of waiting to see whether the body can take care of the infection without medication?

To give you the most information possible, this chapter discusses the role your physician should play in your use of antibiotics, when antibiotics should be used and when they should not be used, and alternative treatments for medical conditions for which antibiotics are frequently prescribed.

Your Physician: A Guide Rather than a Guardian of Your Health

Since medicine is not an exact science but rather an art, and much of the success or failure of a treatment depends on the competency and experience of the physician, it is up to each patient to take an active role in his or her own health care and to become an activated patient. While medical schools and practical experience seek to prepare aspiring doctors for a career in handling illnesses and diseases, much of how a physician attacks and solves problems depends on each physician's attitudes and judgments. Physicians frequently have vastly different opinions on not only how to treat illnesses, but even on what the illness they are treating is. Although doctors are often your best source of information, they may not have all the answers all the time. One example appears below.

A study performed by a Ralph Nader organization called the Center for Science in the Public Interest (CSPI), which puts out a monthly nutrition newsletter, showed just how little some physicians actually know about nutrition. CSPI gave a basic nutrition quiz to physicians with M.D. degrees and to their receptionists. "The results were shocking if not alarming," observed Drs. Schmidt, Smith, and Sehnert. "Nearly all the receptionists passed with flying colors. We won't mention who flunked most of the time!"

What this information proves is that while it is necessary to work with your doctor to reach a diagnosis and determine treatment, it is unwise to place *complete* and sole control of your health in the hands of anyone, including your doctor. "Enter into a health partnership with your doctor rather than surrender your control to the doctor," write Drs. Schmidt, Smith, and Sehnert. This wonderfully sensible statement cannot be emphasized enough when it comes time to deciding whether or not you or your family should take antibiotics.

Your Physician: Helping or Hindering?

Patients are not the only ones who are unaware of the potentially harmful effects of antibiotics; physicians aren't obligated to keep up with the current research in medicine. As stated in *Beyond Antibiotics*:

Doctors usually prescribe antibiotics with sincere motives. That is, they hope the antibiotic will help their patients get well and prevent complications. Obviously, no doctor sets out to intentionally harm patients. Yet doctors have different comfort zones with respect to antibiotics. Some doctors use antibiotics with full awareness of the consequences and restrict their use to only clear indications. Other doctors are somewhat cautious yet quite confident that antibiotics are the solution—thus prescribing them somewhat liberally. Others prescribe them in a somewhat knee-jerk fashion, giving them at the mere hint of something wrong.

What can be done about the lack of physician awareness and acceptance of the serious long-term consequences of antibiotics? Probably not much now, but with warnings from the National Institutes of Health and the CDC, changes are coming. As physicians become more aware of the consequences, they prescribe fewer antibiotics and explain to each patient why in the long run antibiotics may not be good for him.

Physicians and patients respond to the expectations of each other and try to please each other. So even though physicians know antibiotics are unlikely to help, they may give in when patients expect and even demand antibiotics in order to increase patient satisfaction. But hopefully common sense will eventually prevail.

Whether he is unaware of how antibiotics affect our bodies, or unconcerned, or skeptical of the data available depends on each physician's experiences. Despite the research published in medical journals and available for years, some physicians may choose to wait until alternative treatments are fully accepted by mainstream medicine. In an age of widespread litigation and malpractice lawsuits, many physicians may feel it wise to "play it safe" and keep writing prescriptions for infections and ailments. It seems, however, that physicians who are aware of the current research on antibiotics and who are willing to discuss alternatives to antibiotics are through their actions telling their patients that they consider their job to be more than a dispenser of antibiotics and other drugs.

When surveyed, physicians readily admit that they have other reasons for prescribing antibiotics than to aid the patient in recovering from a bacterial infection. A 1989 article in the *Wall Street Journal* reported on a study by Harvard Medical School on the attitudes of physicians who were moderate to heavy prescribers of three drugs:

> Almost half the doctors said they were merely satisfying their patients' demands for these drugs and indicated fears that failure to meet such demands would risk losing

patients to more obliging physicians. Many conceded that the prescribing couldn't be justified on scientific grounds. Another quarter of the doctors cited a placebo effect as justification. Writing a prescription, they argued, can have a positive psychological benefit for the patients and thus possibly bring some relief.

Since working with your physician is crucial to recovering from any serious illness, how can you effectively communicate your desire to avoid antibiotics whenever possible? Drs. Schmidt, Smith, and Sehnert offer several suggestions:

- Do not demand an antibiotic from your physician.

- Ask your physician if anything other than an antibiotic is available, or if waiting a couple of days to see how the infection progresses is a good idea.

- Learn as many medical self-care skills about common infections and medical conditions as possible.

What should you do if your physician thinks you should take antibiotics and, since you have Candida-related problems, you are hesitant to do so? If you have a serious medical condition, such as mitral valve prolapse, taking antibiotics may sometimes be necessary. This brings up another concern: even though you may not be able to start out the journey toward recovery with a physician who is familiar with CRC, it really is necessary to eventually find someone whose judgment you can rely on when questions like this come up.

How Much Is Too Much?

Drs. Schmidt, Smith, and Sehnert offer guidelines so patients can determine whether or not their physician is overprescribing antibiotics. If your physician takes more than five of the following actions, you may be taking antibiotics needlessly or have taken antibiotics needlessly in the past. The recommendations have been divided into three categories to help pinpoint what, if anything, is wrong with the way your physician views antibiotics.

Does your physician prescribe antibiotics without fully investigating the problem?

- Does he prescribe antibiotics after having performed only a brief or cursory examination?

- Does he prescribe antibiotics over the phone?

- Does he prescribe antibiotics without ordering at least a differential blood count?

- Does he grant a refill for an antibiotic prescription without examining you or your child?
- Does he prescribe antibiotics without first addressing your diet and nutritional status?
- Does he prescribe antibiotics without first having done a culture?
- Does he tend to cut short your visit by handing you a prescription and walking out the door?

Does your physician seem to be unaware of the consequences of antibiotics use?

- Does she tell you antibiotics are harmless and do not cause side effects?
- Does she fail to take your concerns about antibiotics safety seriously?
- Does she ignore or discount your descriptions of negative reactions you or your child has had to antibiotics?

Does your physician prescribe antibiotics even when they don't help or when they are unnecessary?

- Does he prescribe antibiotics to a child who is relatively healthy?
- When courses of one or more antibiotics bring no improvement in you or your child, does he simply prescribe more antibiotics?
- Does he prescribe antibiotics when there is a clear indication the infection is not bacterial but rather viral, as in a regular cold?

If your doctor takes *more than five* of these questionable actions, you should bring your concerns to his or her attention and ask to have the situation reassessed. If the physician is unwilling to work with you, find another doctor and make your decision known by walking out. Your health is too important to gamble or take chances with, and that's exactly what you are doing if you stay with a doctor who finds it more convenient to dictate to his or her patients rather than work with them. Any physician intimidated by your questions isn't the one you want helping you regain your health.

Drs. Schmidt, Smith, and Sehnert describe one patient's situation: "One patient, upon bringing her concerns about antibiotics safety to her doctor's attention, was confronted with a gruff 'what medical school did you go to?' Could this doctor be seriously concerned about his patient's welfare? It seems that in such circumstances we believe a change of doctor is in order."

When to Use and When Not to Use Antibiotics

Despite their drawbacks, antibiotics have obviously had an incredibly beneficial impact on society, and no one is suggesting that they be abandoned. In fact antibiotics have been credited with extending the average life ten years. What is being suggested is that they be used wisely, appropriately, and not overused. This is especially important for CRC patients since antibiotics most likely played a part in triggering their initial illness and their use has the ability to hinder recovery.

Just as there is no doubt concerning the myriad benefits of antibiotics, there is also no doubt that antibiotics can negatively affect our bodies in a variety of ways. The most important of these, for our purposes, is antibiotics' tendency to increase Candida growth and suppress immunity.

Drs. Schmidt, Smith, and Sehnert offer six excellent suggestions concerning the correct use of antibiotics:

- Physicians should always perform cultures and sensitivities to determine if bacteria are present and exactly which bacteria are present.

- Tests should be performed to identify which antibiotic would be the most effective against the specific bacteria present.

- The antibiotic with the narrowest spectrum should be used to protect against the elimination of both good and bad bacteria.

- Broad-spectrum antibiotics should be avoided whenever possible. Examples include Keflex, Septra, Bactrim, ampicillin, Ceclor, and amoxicillin.

- The antibiotic should be prescribed for the shortest amount of time possible.

- Nutritional supplements should be recommended whenever infections are present.

There are three considerations to keep in mind when deciding whether or not to use antibiotics. One is whether the infection is acute or chronic, another is whether the person's immune system has been compromised (such as in the case of a potentially fatal disease, such as AIDS), and the third is whether the antibiotics are being used prophylactically, such as during a high-risk surgery or to protect a patient with an abnormal medical condition, such as a heart murmur or mitral valve prolapse.

With acute infections, which often come on rapidly and have severe symptoms, antibiotics are more justified. One extreme example is master puppeteer Jim Henson. He died of acute pneumonia that developed more rapidly than pneumonia generally does. With chronic infections in which antibiotics have been used with little success, however, the use of antibiotics is questionable.

In *Back to Health*, Dr. Remington echoes the need for careful use of antibiotics and advises patients to discuss their concerns with their physicians: "An antibiotic should be used to treat a clear-cut bacterial infection that is potentially dangerous. Tell your doctor you are reluctant to use an antibiotic unless absolutely necessary. He should be willing to work with you, possibly take a culture, or wait a few more days to see how the infection develops. If he feels strongly that you should take treatment, and you agree, then start the antibiotic."

As many CRC patients know, too often well-intentioned physicians are ready to prescribe antibiotics at the slightest hint of infection, even though no danger is apparent. Dr. Remington emphasizes the ability of the body to heal itself: "Many infections are caused by viruses; even if bacterial, many are mild enough that your own immune system can clear them without antibiotics." Whether or not the CRC patient should take an antibiotic depends on the situation. The best answer seems to be "yes" in the case of an acute infection or a medical condition that warrants antibiotics and "no" when it comes to minor ailments that will be cured either without help or with the help of the many natural remedies available at health food stores.

Some antibiotics are worse than others when it comes to causing Candida overgrowth, with the most notorious ones being the powerful broad-spectrum antibiotics. Two antibiotics that generally cause less damage than others are plain penicillin and Erythromycin, and some clinicians recommend them if their use is appropriate for the type of infection present.

Perhaps the best way to protect your body if you have to take an antibiotic is to take nystatin and *Lactobacillus acidophilus* while taking the antibiotic and for one to two weeks after stopping the antibiotic. In chapter 16, several women who have CRC under control report that when they take antibiotics (they had medical conditions or situations that necessitated taking antibiotics), their symptoms resumed. Given this, it is important to explain to your physician your predicament and explore every alternative to antibiotics possible. And if antibiotics are the only solution, remember to take acidophilus at the same time, preferably in a refrigerated powder or pill form available at health food stores.

Antibiotics have been in use over fifty years, since World War II. As more time goes by, however, the more scientists and physicians are realizing that antibiotics are not the only solution, and in fact not even the best solution for many medical conditions. The main reason antibiotics are failing to solve our problems has more to do with the way in which we as a society use antibiotics than the actual properties of antibiotics. In other words, our casual overuse of antibiotics has essentially taken away the effectiveness and option of using antibiotics. Antibiotics should be seen as the last line of defense against most common bacterial diseases, not the first.

Alternatives to Antibiotics

Drugs are unquestionably the backbone of mainstream medicine today. This means that physicians are not encouraged to use other methods; in fact, they are not even taught about alternatives. Physicians can even be censured by colleagues and patients for healing patients with anything other than drugs. One example is a physician who was relieved of his hospital privileges for alleged quackery. As part of his routine surgical procedures the physician would add a few grams of vitamin C to the intravenous fluids of his patients as he was finishing up the operation. The vitamin C helped patients awaken and walk back to their rooms. This particular physician was not censured for failing to help patients, or for even harming patients, but rather for showing enough intelligence to employ a common sense and scientifically proven method of healing.

Recent studies published in medical journals have found several successful, scientifically tested natural alternatives to antibiotics. Given that many of the most effective medications available come from nature (including antibiotics and numerous drugs), it isn't surprising that the future struggle against microbes will involve not antibiotics, but natural elements. As Drs. Schmidt, Smith, and Sehnert point out, "While many Western allopathic doctors would have us believe there is no value to herbal medicine, the evidence shows us otherwise. Seventy-five percent of drugs are based on knowledge of plant substances. One-fourth of all prescription drugs contain one or more plant-derived ingredients." One drug in particular has had a huge impact on childhood leukemia, which once had an 80 percent mortality rate, and now has an 80 percent survival rate. The drug is vincristine and is derived from the rosy periwinkle.

Pure herbs have also been found to be useful against illness. Echinacea, for example, has been used successfully by European doctors to treat upper respiratory infections. Shiitake mushrooms have been proven to hinder viral reproduction and thus slow the development of viral infections. These are just two from a long list of examples. But if these natural substances are so effective and have been scientifically proven, then why aren't their abilities common knowledge? The answer is that since herbal medicines can't be patented, with one company then given exclusive rights to any and all profits, there is not enough incentive for the medical-industrial complex to spend money and time developing them. Plant derivatives, on the other hand, can be manufactured, patented, and sold for huge profits. In addition, the Food and Drug Administration (FDA) is failing to provide incentives for the study of herbal medicines.

Alternative Treatments for Conditions Frequently Treated with Antibiotics

Antibiotics are obviously not the only way to fight infections: a variety of other methods and approaches are not only available, but also very effective. If the infection or the symptoms persist, be sure to see your doctor. However, be aware that in many instances the following medical problems can be taken care of without the help of a physician. If a physician is needed and antibiotics are deemed a good idea, the following treatment methods can be used in conjunction with formal medical treatment.

One of the reasons antibiotics are used instead of alternatives is that alternative treatments usually involve more than just taking pills. They may require lifestyle changes, including taking vitamins and supplements. Some of the more popular medical conditions frequently treated with antibiotics are listed below along with alternative treatments. These conditions are acne, the common cold and influenza, earaches, rhinitis (hay fever), sinusitis, and urinary tract infections (also called bladder infections and cystitis). Many of the remedies listed below help by boosting the immune system. Remember, a weakened immune system, not a chance encounter with a bacterium or virus, is what causes illness.

Acne

Acne is the most common skin disorder, and given that an estimated 80 to 85 percent of adolescents experience disfiguring acne at one time or another, this medical condition should not be taken lightly. Three usual treatments often include an antibiotic, such as tetracycline (Clindamycin) or Retin-A in combination with a topical steroid, and often oral contraceptives.

Since tetracycline, a broad-spectrum antibiotic as described in chapter 5, is frequently and specifically mentioned as a cause of CRC, it should especially be avoided by people with CRC. Tetracyclines were endorsed back in 1969 as proven and acceptable drugs for treatment, but almost ten years later an article in *Lancet* declared the use of antibiotics for acne a "medieval and messy darkness." Of all the antibiotics available, tetracyclines were chosen to treat acne for very practical reasons. Only the tetracyclines seemed to interfere with a certain enzyme produced by propionibacteria, the bacteria that causes acne. Disrupting the enzyme seems to decrease the amount of acne, although the actual cause of acne is unknown.

Unfortunately, all three of the usual treatments are known to cause or contribute to Candida-related problems and are therefore out of the question for people with CRC. So what can be done? Making certain lifestyle and dietary changes has proved extremely effective. Acne is ultimately a result of oils produced by sebaceous glands, which are located in each hair follicle or small area of skin. When the oil becomes trapped, bacteria multiply and the skin becomes inflamed. While no exact cause of acne is known, several factors that contribute are stress, birth control pills, heredity, oily skin, male hormones called androgens (produced during puberty), and allergies.

There are things people with CRC can do to treat acne. Several studies have found zinc to be very helpful. However, the usual amounts used in the research conducted on acne were between 90 and 135mg, an amount that should not be taken without first consulting a physician. According to Drs. Schmidt, Smith, and Sehnert, other treatments that have produced good to excellent results in 92 percent of patients with acne can be divided into two categories: dietary changes and hygienic changes.

Foods and vitamins that should be avoided include: inorganic iron because it inactivates vitamin E; female hormones, such as in birth control pills, because they are also unfriendly to vitamin E; and excess vitamin B_{12} and iodine, which can cause or worsen acne. Other foods that directly worsen acne include: commercial soft drinks that contain brominated vegetable oil and more than one glass of milk per day (the hormones in milk aggravate acne).

Dietary and hygienic changes that will help decrease acne are: taking 50,000 IU (international units) of vitamin A two times a day before meals (consult a physician first); taking 400 IU of vitamin E twice daily before meals; and washing the affected area gently with nonmedicated soap and then applying 5 percent benzoyl peroxide gel or 5 percent tea tree oil gel. Primrose oil has also been used in Europe with good results.

Keeping the area free of oil produced by the skin is also crucial. Two helpful hints are to pat the face with lemon juice three times daily and wash hair frequently. Fifty mg of vitamin B_6 (pyridoxine) taken once or twice a day is also helpful for premenstrual or menstrual acne. If acne persists, remove all dairy products from your diet; the acne may be an allergic reaction to dairy products. Add dairy products back to your diet one at a time to see if acne resumes.

The Common Cold and Influenza

While the common cold and influenza are caused by different microorganisms, the natural remedies for both are similar. The common cold, which is the most common infection in humans, is caused by viruses and not by bacteria. The flu, however is caused by different viruses than the cold. Because of this, antibiotics are useless and should not be given unless bacterial complications, such as pneumonia, arise.

Many physicians justify giving antibiotics by saying they wish to prevent secondary infections, but this form of treatment can lead to superinfections (such as pneumonia) because of increases in antibiotic-resistant bacteria. Symptoms of the common cold include congestion, difficult breathing, headaches, fever, coughing, sneezing, watery eyes, and aches and pains. Because viruses change to adapt to their environment and have hundreds of different forms, colds are hard to cure and developing a vaccine is nearly impossible. Taking the flu shot may not be helpful if a different strain of flu goes around.

When a cold hits, one of the first things people reach for is an over-the-counter medication designed to relieve symptoms. In *Prescription for Nutritional Healing*, James F. Balch, M.D., and Phyllis A. Balch, C.N.C., caution against using nasal decongestants. "Don't use a nasal decongestant to relieve congestion—let the mucus flow. This is the body's way of getting rid of the infection." A recent article in *Medical World News* reports that using over-the-counter medications may actually hinder recovery. According to Drs. Schmidt, Smith, and Sehnert, this is true:

> Antihistamines have been shown to have minimal benefit. Researchers investigating aspirin, ibuprofen and acetaminophen found that all produced 'a significant increase in nasal stuffiness.' Another negative report was that aspirin and acetaminophen suppressed immune function. Cold specialists agree that taking multiple-agent cold preparations is ill-advised. It is better to take one or two with a narrow spectrum of action that matches your symptoms.

If over-the-counter preparations have dubious benefits, then what can be done? There are many natural remedies that can alleviate symptoms and shorten the length of the common cold or flu. In fact, high doses of vitamin C and garlic act as natural antibiotics according to *Alternative Medicine: The Definitive Guide*. Garry F. Gordon, M.D., of Tempe, Arizona, recommends between 10,000 and 20,000mg of vitamin C, divided into three to six doses per day for a

150-pound adult. To help reduce bowel cramping and excessive gas, try using a powdered mineral ascorbate form of vitamin C.

Garlic, which contains allicin, should also be taken along with vitamins A and C. Garlic is a natural antibiotic that also enhances the immune system. Gordon recommends taking either garlic capsules or liquid garlic extract. Both forms provide high doses of allicin and are odor-free. He advises taking ten garlic capsules in the first six hours that you become ill. Some other suggestions include the following:

- To lessen symptoms, take zinc or vitamin C lozenges.
- To shorten the duration of a cold and actually destroy the cold virus, take high doses of one gram per hour of vitamin C.
- To relieve the symptoms of common colds try Perque 1, an amino acid capsule that has met with good clinical success.
- To help relieve symptoms put six drops of eucalyptus oil in a cup of hot water, place a towel over your head, and inhale.

James F. Balch, M.D., and Phyllis A. Balch, C.N.C., recommend a variety of herbs to help alleviate symptoms, including a tea of echinacea, ginger, Pau d'arco (also called Taheebo), yarrow, and slippery elm. For fever they suggest catnip tea enemas and a tincture of 1/4 to 1/2 teaspoon lobelia every three to four hours until the fever drops.

Colds are generally not serious, but if you have the following symptoms or conditions be sure to consult a doctor: if there is congestion in the chest; if your fever goes beyond 102° F for more than three days; if yellow or white spots appear in the throat; if yellow or green mucus is present in the nose or throat; if lymph nodes in the neck and in the jaw become swollen; if chills occur; or if shortness of breath is present.

Earaches

Earaches, also called otitis media or middle ear infections, are the most common reason children are brought to the doctor every year. Earaches often appear after a child has a cold. In fact, nearly 50 percent of earaches in children are preceded by an upper respiratory infection such as a cold, and not surprisingly, the most common complication of a cold in children is a middle ear inflammation. Eighty percent of children will have at least one ear infection during their first five years.

Ear infections happen when the eustachian tube in the ear becomes blocked and infected. Diagnosis is not based on symptoms, but rather on examination of the eardrum using an otoscope, which examines the outer and middle ear. Electronic monitoring of the eardrum is also a dependable method that is frequently used. It is extremely important that middle ear problems in children be treated and taken very seriously. According to Drs. Schmidt, Smith, and Sehnert, "Hearing loss, intellectual impairment, and delays in language development can occur when middle ear problems are long-standing."

Earaches are usually treated with antibiotics, and antibiotics prescribed for earaches account for 42 percent of the antibiotics given to children every year. This figure is high given the startling news that bacteria may not even be the cause of the earache. Drs. Schmidt, Smith, and Sehnert quote recent research on otitis media and write: "Experts point out that 30 to 50 percent of painful middle ears contain no bacteria. Antibiotics would be of little use in such children. Moreover, up to 70 percent of children who have been unresponsive to antibiotic therapy or surgery have no bacteria in their middle ears."

Then what is the cause of their middle ear problems? Several causes of earaches have been identified and include food allergies, especially dairy products such as milk and cheese. Other contributors are a diet high in dietary fats, which can cause inflammation of the middle ear, and deficiencies in zinc and vitamin A, which can change middle ear cells and lead to buildup of fluid in the ear. The rate of ear infections also seems to be higher in the homes of smokers.

It is doubtful that these problems, along with bacteria, are the only causes of otitis media, but since bacteria doesn't seem to be the main culprit, it makes even more sense to be careful with antibiotics. Recurrent childhood earaches not only have many causes but, as previously mentioned, can also be extremely critical. If your child has a serious problem with earaches, one book that may be able to help is *Childhood Ear Infections: What Every Parent and Physician Should Know About Prevention, Home Care, and Alternative Treatment* by Dr. Michael A. Schmidt and published by North Atlantic Books.

As with other medical conditions in which antibiotics are frequently prescribed, not only have antibiotics been shown to not always help the situation, but they can actually do harm. One common problem with treating earaches with broad-spectrum antibiotics is that yeast/fungal infections of the middle ear can occur. Even more alarming is recent research indicating that antibiotics may lead to recurrent ear infections in children. An article in the *Journal of the American Medical Association* reports that children who were given amoxicillin for chronic earaches had two to six times more recurrent ear problems than children who had not been treated with antibiotics.

Several natural and common sense treatments, however, are available to treat ear infections. Dr. Fred Pullen, an ear, nose, and throat specialist in Florida, found that 75 percent of children who had recurrent ear problems stopped having them when dairy products were taken away. Additional food allergies may also be responsible or may contribute to the problem. One common sense preventative method is to breast-feed your baby for as long as possible. According to *Alternative Medicine: The Definitive Guide*, "Recent studies show that the longer a baby is nursed, the less likely he or she will be able to contract otitis media and other infections." Other studies have suggested that breast milk boosts the natural immunity of the child and that it contains natural nutrients such as *Lactobacillus acidophilus*. Other remedies include the following:

- Avoiding all processed foods, including refined sugar.
- Increasing the good bacteria in the body. Infants can be given bifidus or acidophilus supplements, and children should be given acidophilus. Two immune system boosters, echinacea and garlic oil capsules, are also an excellent idea.
- Boosting the immune system by increasing the amount of vitamin C in the diet to 1,000mg three times a day. Fifteen mg of zinc can be given each day, although it is best not to take this amount of zinc for more than several weeks. Ask your physician.
- Trying homeopathic remedies available at your health food store.

Rhinitis (Hay Fever)

Allergic rhinitis, commonly known as hay fever, is suspected to affect as many as one in ten people in the United States. Although it is often triggered by pollen and other environmental factors, rhinitis is actually a disorder of the immune system. The immune system is responsible for recognizing the difference between intruders to the body and nonharmful substances. Allergic reactions to dust, pollen, and other substances mean that the immune system is interpreting harmless substances as threatening and then attacking them.

Although allergic symptoms are frequently treated with antihistamines or antibiotics, they can be relieved naturally. One of the most effective methods of controlling allergies, including hay fever, is to change the diet to include foods that decrease mucus and to exclude foods known to cause allergic reactions.

Foods that may help combat rhinitis are in general high-fiber, whole foods, including noncitrus fruits, vegetables, nuts, and raw seeds. Grains are another food that can help fight rhinitis, although not all CRC patients can tolerate them. Raw (uncooked) juices, especially carrot, beet, spinach, celery, and parsley, are also helpful. Nutritional supplements that also provide relief are evening primrose oil, 50 to 80mg of zinc (unless you have a fever), 100mg three times daily of vitamins B_5 (pantothenic acid), 50mg of B_6 (pryidoxine) two times daily, vitamins A, C, and E, and MaxEPA, an essential fatty acid. Other supplements that have been reported to ease symptoms and promote healing are bee pollen, royal jelly capsules (as directed on label), 100mg of germanium twice daily, 500mg twice daily of raw thymus glandulars, and 30mg of coenzyme Q_{10} two times per day.

Many people who have respiratory allergies are also allergic to a variety of foods. You may be allergic to all, some, or none of the following foods, and the best way to find out is to perform a self-test by eliminating them from your diet and then reintroducing the foods one at a time. Foods widely known to cause allergies should be avoided. They are dairy products, wheat, peanuts, eggs, chocolate, and shellfish. It is also a good idea to eliminate caffeine, tobacco, sugar, and alcohol from your diet if you haven't already. Artificial food additives, including preservatives and especially food colorings, should also be avoided.

Sinusitis

Sinusitis, or inflammation of the sinuses, affects about two million people and is one of the most common health problems in America today. Although sinusitis is universal, that does not mean it should be taken lightly. If you notice any swelling around the eyes, immediately contact your physician. Untreated sinus problems can lead to serious respiratory disorders including pneumonia, asthma, and bronchitis.

About 50 percent of sinusitis is caused by bacteria, which is one reason antibiotics are frequently prescribed. Although it is less common, viruses and mold can also cause sinusitis. Candida is the cause of many cases of sinusitis, while dental abscesses are responsible for 10 to 15 percent of adult cases of sinusitis. Allergies to airborne substances and indoor pollutants are also frequently responsible for episodes of sinusitis.

Symptoms are usually sinus pain, earaches, toothaches, headaches, congestion, fever, malaise, and nasal discharge. Sinus pain can become worse when the patient bends over. Sinus problems are also known to follow upper respiratory infections. Adults have sinusitis more often than children.

One way to treat sinusitis is to first treat what may be causing sinus irritation: hay fever or colds. One widely used natural sinus remedy is the herb *Ephedra sinica,* although it should be avoided during pregnancy. *Ephedra sinica* is often used in conjunction with *Echinacea purpurea,* goldenseal root, and ginger root. Other natural remedies include the following:

- Drinking hot liquids because they help mucus flow.
- Taking 50,000 IU of beta carotene and 6,000mg of vitamin C daily.
- Taking 50mg of zinc per day and 400 IU of vitamin E per day.
- Avoiding the use of topical decongestants (nasal sprays) for more than three or four days because they can prolong symptoms.
- Avoiding foods known to cause food allergies (they are listed in the rhinitis section).
- Avoiding airborne allergens that can aggravate symptoms. Some are dander from pets, pollen, dust, and cigarette smoke.

A variety of natural supplements are available to help people who suffer from chronic sinusitis. They include 200 micrograms of selenium per day, one or two grams of bioflavonoids per day, and 500 micrograms of N-acetyl cysteine per day. Essential fatty acids, such as evening primrose oil, black currant oil, flaxseed oil, and vitamin B_5, are also very important.

Urinary Tract Infections (Bladder Infections or Cystitis)

Urinary tract infections (UTIs) affect about twenty-five million American women every year, but are rare in men under age forty. In men over forty, UTIs often indicate inflammation of the prostate gland. An estimated one in five women will have a UTI at least once in her life, and some women will have UTIs more than once. UTIs are also responsible for 5.2 million doctor's office visits per year and an estimated one billion dollars in health-care expenses. Girls under age two can also get UTIs from improper wiping after a bowel movement because this carries fecal bacteria into the urethra.

UTIs occur when bacteria get inside the urinary tract and multiply, resulting in an infection that causes discomfort. A full 70 percent of infections are caused by the common intestinal bacteria *E. coli.* Fortunately UTIs are rarely serious, except in pregnant women or in women who have recurrent UTIs (generally defined as developing a UTI a few weeks after being treated for one).

Women who are more prone to this problem fall among the following categories: sexually active, sexually active with multiple partners, pregnant, women who had UTIs as children, women who have had diabetes, and women who are past menopause. Several things can cause UTIs, including sexual intercourse, waiting too long to urinate, antibiotics, and spermicidal preparations, such as those containing nonoxynol-9.

Symptoms first start when the woman has a strong urge to urinate that cannot be postponed. When urine is released, the woman feels a sharp pain or burning sensation and very little urine is eliminated. The urine may also be tinged with blood. This cycle may also repeat itself over several days. Soreness may be present in the back, sides, or lower abdomen. Given that most people urinate about six times a day, to urinate more frequently could indicate a UTI.

UTIs can become complicated if the bacteria spread to the ureters and then to the kidneys, and additional symptoms of back pain, chills, nausea, fever, and vomiting may result in addition to the symptoms already listed. An estimated one hundred thousand patients are hospitalized with UTIs every year. Since the common symptoms associated with them are common to many problems, it is important that you consult a doctor before treating yourself for a UTI. Your physician can perform several tests that will either confirm or deny an infection.

Another reason to speak to your doctor is that an estimated five hundred thousand women who have symptoms of UTIs may have interstitial cystitis (IC), which is a chronic inflammation of the bladder. IC is not responsive to either natural or antibiotic treatments. Food allergy, however, seems to be a frequent contributor. Your physician can determine if you have IC by performing a cystoscopy, a test in which the inside of the urethra and bladder are examined. According to an article by Dr. Crook in *Health Line*, a newsletter formerly put out by Dr. Crook's International Health Foundation, some women with IC have had success in getting rid of the problem by taking Diflucan and following a sugar-free diet.

Customary treatment includes a variety of antibiotics, however, there are many easy ways to prevent UTIs and treat them naturally once they occur:

- Practice good hygiene by washing the skin around the rectum, vagina, and the area in between every day and before and after you have intercourse.
- After urination or bowel movement, wipe from front to back to decrease the chances bacteria will get into the urinary tract.
- Drink plenty of fluids to clear bacteria out of your urinary system.
- Urinate as soon as you feel the urge, or every two or three hours. It is also a good idea to urinate before and after sex to help empty out bacteria that may enter the urethra during intercourse.

- Wear panties with a cotton crotch because cotton doesn't trap moisture near the skin.

- Eliminate the following foods and additives known to aggravate the bladder from your diet: tea, coffee, caffeine, artificial sweeteners, tomato-based foods, and carbonated beverages.

Perhaps the best known natural remedy for UTIs is cranberry juice. It has been found to be very effective in treating, but not always preventing UTIs. Although for many years the use of cranberry juice was dismissed as being simple folklore wisdom, recent studies cited in a letter to the editor in the *New England Journal of Medicine* provide insight into why cranberry juice works: both cranberry and blueberry juice have an ingredient that keeps bacteria from sticking to or invading the lining cells of the bladder.

One problem, however, is that most brands of commercial cranberry juice contain only about 10 percent actual cranberry juice. The addition of sugar, which is often included, can counteract the beneficial effects of the cranberry juice. Fortunately, there are other options besides cranberry juice cocktails from your supermarket. Cranberry juice can be purchased in both pure 100 percent juice form or in supplement form. Walnut Acres in Pennsylvania sells a juice that is 100 percent cranberry. Their address is Penns Creek, PA 17862; phone number, (800) 433-3998. The supplement is called Crangel and contains 3,000mg of concentrated cranberry juice power, which is the equivalent of eight ounces of pure cranberry juice. The supplement can either be purchased at your local health food store or by contacting Nutrition Dynamics, Maple Plain, MN 55359; phone number, (800) 444-9998. Along with cranberry or blueberry juice, be sure to take vitamin C and bioflavonoids at the same time because they work synergistically to enhance the effectiveness of both juices.

Other natural remedies for UTIs include the following:

- Make sure you get enough vitamin C, either through your diet or by taking vitamin C supplements. Recommended dosages range from 3,000 to 8,000mg daily. Vitamin C makes urine acidic, which reduces the amount of harmful bacteria. However, in chronic cases, vitamin C has been found to be irritating in doses of over one to two grams. You can also try taking one-half teaspoon of baking soda or two Alka-Seltzer Gold tablets.

- Take 30 to 50mg of vitamin B_1 two or three times a day in between meals for no more than one week to help reduce pain, irritation, and burning.

Drs. Schmidt, Smith, and Sehnert also offer several recommendations to treat UTIs. In addition to taking pure cranberry products as
noted above, try taking acidophilus; 5,000 IU of vitamin A; 50,000
IU of beta carotene; or *Cantharis*, a homeopathic medicine, which
should be taken three times a day.

All of these medical conditions discussed in this chapter have at
least one thing in common: like CRC, they are all results of a weakened immune system. Many of the suggestions listed under each section are aimed at boosting the immune system so it can better fight
illness. Your immune system is your best protection against any and
all bacteria, viruses, and other potentially harmful medical conditions and diseases. So keep your immune defenses healthy by getting
the proper amount of rest, following the Candida control diet,
drinking plenty of liquids, taking daily supplements, avoiding stress,
and in general just taking care of yourself.

—16—

Advice from Men and Women Who Have CRC

Experience is the mother of truth; and by experience we learn wisdom.
—William Shippen, Jr., quoted by Betsy C. Corner in *William Shippen, Jr.*

Case histories are more than who, what, when, and where; they are real people with real lives and real problems. In this chapter thirteen unique individuals, both men and women, share their experiences with CRC and the wisdom they've gleaned from those experiences. They have different needs and have found different ways to meet them. With their own voices and in their own words, these patients describe their illnesses and offer insight into what has helped them most.

The questions contained in these interviews were designed to help people with CRC relate to and understand the experiences of these thirteen patients and to alleviate some of the isolation CRC patients often experience. Because CRC, like many chronic illnesses, affects the entire life of each patient, some of the questions go beyond medical information and give you a glimpse into the personal lives of these CRC patients and how they have resolved the everyday problems that arise.

The patients who participated in these interviews share many similar characteristics. They have taken control of their health and have realized that they can no longer solely depend on health professionals to monitor and determine their good health. They are also more appreciative of their health and actively work to gain and then to keep it. Before their illness began, many were so busy taking care of others they forgot to take care of themselves. That changed; in their responses to the questions that follow many emphasized new respect and attention to their own lives and needs.

These patients are in different stages of illness. One was very recently diagnosed, many are still sick, most have their CRC under control, and others are getting better or completely well. Although they are all different, many share similar characteristics. For example, several mentioned that they now realize they have had Candida their entire lives. And three, Johanna, Kristy, and Roger, have both CRC and CFS. Please allow me to introduce Blair, Beverly, Dora, Deborah, Jonathon, Johanna, Kristy, Marla, Megan, Mary Jo, Natalie, Pauline, and Roger:

Blair is thirty years old and stays at home with her three young children. During the day she also takes care of other children in her home. She has been sick since 1982 and continues to look for solutions to her CRC. Blair is originally from Michigan and presently lives in Arkansas. Her health problems began shortly after her marriage when she began taking birth control pills, and her CRC severely complicated all three of her pregnancies. Although Blair is presently feeling better, she still hasn't recovered.

Beverly described herself as a fifty-seven-year-old grandmother who is now retired from her job because of her CRC. She is originally from Arkansas and now lives in Michigan. She was exposed to Candida through her job in a hospital, an environment known to have high rates of infections from Candida. Her most persistent symptoms were soreness and pain in her legs and hands, and hypertension. Although she retired early from her job at the hospital, she said except for her allergies she is feeling much better. "I have been having these problems now for about fifteen years, but I am getting better after I started seeing an environmental doctor and doing lots of self-help things," she said.

Dora is originally from Pennsylvania and currently lives in New York state. She is forty-six years old, and in addition to having Candida she also has mitral valve prolapse. What triggered her CRC was exposure to pesticides at the senior housing complex in which she worked. Her most persistent symptoms are her chemical sensitivities which she still suffers from today. Because of her severe reactions to personal-care products she very rarely leaves her house.

Deborah is seventy-seven years old and described herself as a happily married housewife with four successful children, seven grandchildren, and eight great-grandchildren. She has lived in Michigan her entire life and estimates that she has had Candida for twenty-five to thirty years and is still fighting it. Her CRC was brought on by antibiotics and a high-sugar diet.

Jonathon has either been a pharmacist or been around pharmacists his entire life. As a child he grew up in a pharmacy surrounded by his uncles and fathers who were all pharmacists. During his childhood, everyone he knew would be either a pharmacist or a doctor. He is from California originally and graduated from Columbia University with a degree in pharmacy. Jonathon, now fifty-two, runs a pharmacy/ health food store. He developed CRC from using large amounts of antibiotics as a child and has had CRC since 1985.

Johanna is forty-five years old and has lived in southeastern Michigan for most of her life. She was diagnosed as having both CRC and CFS only six weeks before her interview. She said she felt both frustrated and isolated. Johanna said she wasn't working but instead was concentrating on getting better.

Kristy, forty-one, is happily married with three children. Kristy's family is extremely important to her, and she was very upset by her illness because it prevented her from taking care of them. She said she takes care of everyone but has difficulty letting anyone take care of her. She had a very upbeat attitude about her health even though after ten years she still isn't completely well. Kristy doesn't just have CRC, she also has CFS, and she thinks maybe another undiagnosed health problem that is keeping her from regaining her health. She works out of her home office with her husband running an international marketing business. She is glad to have this opportunity because she said given her health problems she would not be able to keep a job outside her home.

Marla, in her sixties, is from Virginia originally and now lives in New York state. She has a degree in education and has worked part-time in libraries. While her health is satisfactory at the moment, because of the possibility that she has a heart murmur, Marla sometimes has to take antibiotics, which cause a flare-up of symptoms. She has found nystatin and acidophilus to be very helpful. When asked if she thinks CRC will ever be accepted by the medical community she declared, "It will take an announcement from Harvard or Yale."

Megan is originally from a large city in upstate New York. She described herself as forty-three years old and happily married. She is also a mother of two young children and currently expecting her third child. She is very involved in her son's school and in community work in general. Although she is now a stay-at-home mother, she has worked in several job fields including real estate and broadcast news. Her CRC was caused by several factors, including exposure to chemicals, antibiotics, and pesticides. Although she was sick for five and a half years, she said she has completely recovered from CRC.

Mary Jo is from New Jersey originally and currently lives in New York state. She described herself as looking younger than her actual age: "I'm sixty-one, but I look forty-five." She is a technical illustrator and has also done office work. She has had CRC for about two years and is steadily recovering. Her CRC was caused by antibiotics and stress, and her symptoms included depression, panic attacks, vaginitis, and insomnia.

Natalie described herself as a tall, skinny, active woman in her mid-forties. She is from Pennsylvania originally and said the worst years of her illness occurred from 1978 to 1986. She has been well for five years. Although she didn't have as severe a case of CRC as other people who have experienced it, she found it very hard to cope with her unexplainable symptoms.

Pauline is thirty-six years old, originally from Arkansas, and a housewife and homemaker. She helps her husband, an engineer, with his business and home schools their two children, a son and a daughter. "I never felt I could hold down a full-time job—partially because of the way I was raised, I have always felt I should be at home taking care of things," she said. She was very educated and informed about CRC. At first, Pauline resisted going on the anti-Candida diet and treating her CRC. She said that at the time, she hoped that her health problems would just go away.

Roger is forty-six years old, from Ohio originally, and now lives in Florida. He has both CRC and CFS. He said his two major interests are health in general and CRC. "Candida is a magnification of a lot of illnesses people have suffered from for a long time," he said. Roger also describes himself as having both a type A and a codependent personality and as having a tendency to focus on one area so much he loses track of other things. Roger has a master's degree in engineering and works as a civil engineer.

One of the most distinct features of CRC is that although similarities can be found in each medical history, everyone who has CRC has his or her own unique struggle with it. Blair, Beverly, Dora, Deborah, Jonathon, Johanna, Kristy, Marla, Megan, Mary Jo, Natalie, Pauline, and Roger are no exception. All had their lives affected in a wide variety of ways, and all had different symptoms and experiences.

Please describe your experiences with Candida, including your most persistent symptoms and when they started.

Blair   Although Blair's symptoms started when she took birth control pills, her most striking and alarming experiences with Candida involved her severe problems with all three of her pregnancies. Her experiences with pregnancy contributed to her declining health, and after the births of her children, she had flare-ups of symptoms.

In 1985, when she was twenty, she gave birth to her first child, who was born two months premature. Since the baby was in a breach position, he was delivered by cesarean section. The next few months were very hard on Blair and wore down her health in general. Since her new son slept very little, Blair was up with him many nights. At that time, she was also given antibiotics for postpartum depression. "I really went through a tough time after he was born." Around this time, she began experiencing headaches, mood swings, irritability (including a short temper), and depression. In addition to her history of constipation and vaginal yeast infections, she also had eczema on her hands. She went to several physicians who told her she was just tired and attributed her symptoms to the fact that she had just delivered a baby.

During this time she and her husband were having financial problems because of the new baby. The financial problems were in part due to the fact that although the new baby was covered by their family health insurance, they did not have maternity insurance and Blair's health problems were becoming expensive. It would still be six years before Blair realized she had CRC.

In 1988 Blair became pregnant again. "I had just started

feeling better!" she lamented. She had started a strict diet to try to improve her health. The diet was similar to the Candida control diet, and it had helped her somewhat.

With her second pregnancy she had severe morning sickness, and the nausea was so intense she couldn't work. "With my second [pregnancy] it was even worse; I vomited to the point of dehydration." She started premature labor when the baby was only eighteen weeks old. Over the course of the pregnancy, she was in the hospital ten times for premature labor and similar problems. For both her second and third pregnancies, she was on medication designed to halt premature labor. For the last six weeks of her second pregnancy, her doctor prescribed total bed rest and would let her get up only to go to the bathroom.

Blair's second child, a daughter, was born at thirty-six weeks, one month premature. She and the baby went home the next day, but after four days, the baby turned yellow. Both mother and daughter went back to the hospital and were given a private room, and Blair was solely responsible for caring for the child twenty-four hours a day, which included feeding the baby every two hours. This lasted seven days. "That was when the blues hit," she said. During this time, she was never able to rest and had very little help from the hospital staff.

After she had her second child, her CRC symptoms worsened and she had severe mental problems, mood swings, and even worse vaginal problems. She describes herself as being in a mental fog and as not being able to remember anything. Her memory problems were so severe she even forgot to feed her new daughter. She started another diet to lose weight and started feeling better.

As with her second pregnancy, in 1990 when Blair started feeling better, she became pregnant again. And as with the other two pregnancies, after she had the baby her symptoms increased and intensified. But this time was different. Her health became much worse. She said, "By this time I'd really stirred things up." Thankfully, it was soon after this third severe flare-up of symptoms that she learned about CRC from a friend.

She was extremely sick and nauseous for the first three months of this pregnancy. She took premature labor medication until the thirty-sixth week, when her doctor discontinued the medication because she had been put on an antibiotic, Keflex, for strep throat for ten days. The day after she discontinued the premature labor medication Blair gave birth to her third child.

Because of the Keflex, Blair kept getting infections, including sinus and pelvic infections. She also experienced a return of her previous symptoms (which had stopped when she went on the strict diet) and her sugar cravings began. Although she tried to eat nutritiously, she snacked on nonnutritious food.

Beverly   During the first year she worked at the hospital, Beverly started having respiratory problems and other unexplainable symptoms. "One year from the day I was hired, I was hospitalized with what was said to be asthma. I was put on breathing medication, but my health problems kept multiplying. I had chest pains, fluid on the knee, sore throats, hypersensitivity, and hypertension. The medications that were given to me only made me worse. Sometimes I thought I was getting better, and the symptoms would come back worse than before."

Beverly described her most persistent symptoms as soreness and pain in her legs and hands and hypertension. "It got to the point where I could hardly get up and out of a chair. These symptoms started after the doctor I was seeing gave me a flu shot. A week later, I started having numbness in my right hand and foot and also pain. I was told I had arthritis and Lyme disease."

Dora   After being exposed to pesticides, Dora lost her hearing and had a constant, sharp pain in one eye. Right now, she feels sick and gets headaches whenever she comes in contact with chemicals. She also had severe and continuous headaches for five years. Currently, things that always trigger her symptoms are after-shave and clothes that have been washed or dried with fabric softener. She also reacts to fertilizers, cigarette smoke, and perfume. "Perfume is poison," she said. "I'm not as bad as some people. I was sensitive to milk and yeast, but I had no problems with molds. It was mainly chemicals."

Deborah   Deborah said she has been sick with Candida between twenty-five and thirty years. Her symptoms were a result of incomplete digestion. "I had a nonmalignant tumor under my spinal cord removed in 1977. After that, I had many years of gas—I burped after every meal—and I recently found I wasn't making any hydrochloric acid, so I wasn't absorbing nutrients from my foods or supplements." Her most persistent symptoms were dizziness, sore muscles and muscle mass loss, feelings of disorientation, gastric problems, and lack of energy.

Jonathon   Although he always had allergies, Jonathon developed asthma in July or August 1985 and became ill with CRC the same year after having surgery for nasal polyps. To this day, he doesn't know exactly what triggered his CRC. "All of a sudden I got very sick." He was paralyzed from his diaphragm down and hospitalized numerous times. "I was dying. One neurologist looked at me, figured I had AIDS, and wouldn't even touch me."

No one knew what was wrong with him. "The diagnosis was that, basically, my nervous system was coming apart at the seams." It would be three years before he would find out what was wrong. During that time, he was confined to his bed and coughed up pounds of mucus every day. He didn't realize it at the time but everything he was eating was killing him. Because of the three years in bed, Jonathon had muscle atrophy and in order to recover had to go through physical therapy.

Johanna   Johanna had always had some chemical sensitivities and depression, but said her symptoms became much worse a year ago. "Lately it seems like it's been one thing after another. I've always had a lot of depression and anxiety all my life, or for at least as long as I can remember. Whether or not they're related [to the Candida] I don't know."

Before she was diagnosed with CRC, she went to the allergy department of a large local university health facility, and they told her they had no idea what she had. "It makes me so angry. I spent so much time and money, and they basically wrote me off."

Johanna's symptoms are mostly extreme chemical sensitivities, and she can't go near petroleum products, especially inks. She said soy-based inks, Xerox inks, and computer inks cause the worst discomfort and pain. Because of her sensitivities, she can't be near any form of reading material. In addition to inks, Johanna can't tolerate plastics, perfumes, deodorants, or smoking. She also experiences chronic fatigue, which she said makes her feel "burned out" all the time.

Kristy   When her symptoms first started, Kristy thought she had the flu; she would be sick for a few days every couple of weeks. Then her sick periods began to be longer and longer. Her symptoms would vary from time to time, but throughout her illness she always has had extreme fatigue. She also had blurred vision. Although she had a regular temperature, she felt feverish. She also had two other frequently reported symptoms: short-term memory loss and not being able to think straight. For the last few years, she has had a lot of gastrointestinal symptoms, such as gas, bloating, and cramps. As a result, she has to be very careful what she eats.

Over the ten years of her illness, Kristy said, the course of her health can be divided into three categories. For the first seven years she was extremely sick and very limited in what she could do. When describing that time in her life, she said she would be in bed for one or two weeks at a time. She said she also completely lacked energy. "I actually had to lie there and think about whether or not I could pick up a glass of water." During this time she also had periods of five or six months when she would be symptom-free.

The second and third stages mark her progression toward improved health. Kristy said when she finished her initial treatments about three years ago, her health turned around. The third, and so far final, stage began a year and a half ago when she underwent a treatment called colonic irrigation, which is a method of cleaning out the large intestine. She credits colonic irrigation with improving her health by 50 percent.

Marla   About forty years ago, while Marla was in college, she had a cyst at the tip of her spine removed and was given sulfa drugs. After the sulfa drugs, she remembers having overall feelings of unwellness, not feeling right, not being able to concentrate, and having a problem with fungus around her fingernails. She continued to have problems for about a year, and then the symptoms stopped.

Around 1982, she said, she noticed depression immediately after haven taken antibiotics and after having her thyroid pills adjusted. Her other symptoms included gas, various digestive problems, vaginitis, and severe itchy scalp/skin problems. She currently has problems with low blood sugar. She is suspected of having a heart murmur and is given antibiotics periodically as a precautionary measure. Whenever she has to take them, her symptoms resume or increase.

Megan   Megan was sick about five and a half years, from the time when she was thirty-four until she was thirty-nine. "It got better as the years went on. I inched toward health and held that line, rarely going back." Getting a correct diagnosis took about a year and a half, and like many patients Megan became worse immediately after the diagnosis.

Megan's most persistent symptoms were fatigue, panic attacks and extreme, daily headaches. She later developed arthritis and asthma. She also had chemical sensitivities, which she describes as fleeting, but she had trouble figuring out exactly which chemicals or synthetic materials were making her sick whenever she felt sensitivities. "My health was too clouded. There were too many issues I had to work on at that time." She said she had both physical and mental problems, with one of the more persistent mental issues being unresolved anger that started over financial problems.

Megan's severe headaches disappeared completely within a week of her changing her diet. The other symptoms subsided after a few months.

Mary Jo

Mary Jo's CRC began two years ago, and she said that at the time she didn't know her symptoms were connected to each other and a single illness. She described herself as very nervous and jumpy and said she also had terrible insomnia, joint pains, panic attacks, severe headaches, depression, irritable bowels, and sugar cravings. "I couldn't get enough sugar or starch; all I was hungry for was sugar and starch. I now realize I was feeding the Candida beasties."

Mary Jo also had vaginal yeast infections even though she'd never had vaginal problems before. She said she could feel her blood pressure going up for no apparent reason, and one time she had an anxiety attack and chest pains and called an ambulance. The emergency medical technicians told her she was at the point of having a stroke. When she arrived at the hospital tests showed her heart to be in perfect condition. "The anxiety attacks were the final straw, as you might say, that broke the camel's back."

Natalie

Natalie was sick from 1978 until 1986, when she found out she had CRC. "I struggled along, yet I knew something wasn't right. It's kind of hard to pinpoint it; I just didn't feel right. It wasn't something I could live with."

Initially, she had vaginal infections and later developed depression, a reduced mental capacity, and inability to concentrate. She also had pains in her legs and sides, aches in her neck and legs, and a ringing noise in both her ears.

Pauline

Pauline's symptoms started after taking birth control pills as a teenager and continued for the next twelve years. She mainly had digestive problems, including diarrhea, nausea, intestinal problems, bloating, and constipation. In addition, she had an ulcer and was diagnosed as having a spastic colon. She found her symptoms were all related to her menstrual cycle. Also, when her CRC was worse she had more menstrual problems, including cramps during periods.

"I can remember when I started feeling better, I had more energy. I felt so much better than I did then that I got involved in a lot of projects around the house." Pauline said getting well affected her emotionally and helped her relationship with her family and husband.

But, unfortunately, her health problems resumed. After feeling better for a time, she and her family moved into a house in which smokers had previously lived and which also had a mold problem, and her health became worse. At that time, she had to watch her diet even more closely.

Roger   "Eight or nine years ago I could do whatever I wanted and always recover," Roger said. His worst symptoms were overriding fatigue, food allergies, floaters in his eyes, problems with his GI tract, and hypoglycemia. "My hypoglycemia—that was the worst," he said. Another disastrous symptom was his mental fogginess. "My ability to think and concentrate was greatly affected. It got to the point where I couldn't work out anymore."

He cited fatigue, lack of endurance, and muscle pain as why he had to stop weightlifting. "It's crazy how my Candida makes my CFS worse. I think they're the same thing."

For everyone but Beverly and Deborah, antibiotics or birth control pills (or a combination of both) caused or added to their CRC. Other contributing factors were emotional/physical stress, pesticides, and a poor diet.

What caused your Candida-related problems?

Blair   As a child, Blair said, she was on "lots and lots" of antibiotics. Although before she married she was having mild forms of the symptoms that would later characterize her CRC, her symptoms greatly intensified when she began taking birth control pills shortly after her marriage. "After I got married, it all went downhill. They really threw it [my health] into orbit. If I hadn't had the birth control pills, I never would have gotten this bad."

Beverly   "It was only in 1978 when I took a job working in housekeeping at a medical hospital that I became ill," said Beverly. "I found out later that Candida can be passed on from hand to hand by hospital workers and also that it is found in hospitals. I was given this information by a medical epidemiologist. I am sure I got this from working at that hospital."

Dora   Although Dora said she did have antibiotics for ear infections as a child, what triggered her CRC was overexposure to pesticides at the senior housing complex where she worked. She said the management at the senior housing complex chemically exterminated inside the building and used lawn chemicals outside. "People just don't get it; they just really wanted a green lawn."

Deborah   "I think maybe my diet of coffee, sugar, white flour, antibiotics, and stress [caused my CRC]," Deborah said. Her physicians gave her penicillin for the phlebitis she developed when she delivered her last child. Phlebitis is inflammation of the walls of a vein, often in the leg.

Jonathon   Because of his infections and allergies, Jonathon was given large doses of antibiotics. When penicillin, the first antibiotic, first came out during World War II, it was available only to the military. Despite this, as a pharmacist, Jonathon's father had access to black market penicillin and the newest and latest antibiotics as they were coming out. "We got them and we got them fast," Jonathon said. No one thought twice about giving Jonathon antibiotics. His ear infections were not only serious but also the kind known to cause deafness. "There was a good reason to use antibiotics," he said.

At the time an article in a popular magazine was written about the high amounts of antibiotics Jonathon had been given for his infections, more antibiotics in fact than anyone else. "When I was four years old I'd been on antibiotics more than anyone alive."

Jonathon was also given high doses of antibiotics prophylactically over many years. For example, as a child he was given one million units of penicillin every day for two years by injection. At the same time, he was also given large amounts of antihistamines and decongestants for his allergies.

Johanna   Johanna reports that she took birth control pills off and on from age twenty to thirty. "Mostly on," she adds. "From what I've read that's probably the culprit." Around the time she became really sick she was working in the food industry, and the plastic products around her contributed to her illness.

Kristy   Kristy said she ate a very poor diet and has a history of antibiotic use. She also described herself as having a type A personality and said she puts a great deal of stress on herself to get too much done. "I fell into the same trap a lot of women have. I tried to do too much. I tried to be superwoman."

Marla   Marla believes antibiotics caused her Candida-related problems.

Megan   Megan's CRC was caused by a wide variety of factors, including exposure to chemicals, birth control pills, a history of antibiotics and topical corticosteroid medications, and exposure to pesticides. Stress from her active and demanding jobs also contributed. She described herself before CRC as being "highly motivated to do well in business."

Before her present marriage, Megan was married to a physician and had unlimited access to antibiotics, and she took them frequently. "I had them throughout my life for every stupid little thing."

When Megan married at twenty-one, she went on the pill, which gave her a "false state of well-being." When she was on the pill, all her allergies left her and she felt great. She was on the pill for eight years until she decided it was prudent to get off. After she stopped taking birth control pills, she had all four of her wisdom teeth removed and developed an infection for which she was given antibiotics for about two months. She also began to get unexplainable cases of hives. "From that time on, things slid downhill," she said.

Besides antibiotics and birth control pills, Megan was also exposed to chemicals when she bought and renovated a new house. She also applied pesticides to the yard. "That's what started this," she said. She completely restored the house, including having it painted inside and having new plastering, carpeting, and furnishings. "I crashed," she said. "My health just plummeted. Part was the pesticides, part of it was the renovation of the new house, my new car, and renovations at work."

Mary Jo   Mary Jo suspects that what started her CRC was the antibiotics she was given for several serious illnesses. Three and a half years ago she had mycoplasma pneumonia, also called walking pneumonia, a contagious disease with symptoms of coughing, fever, and other signs of upper respiratory infection, which is frequently treated with antibiotics. One year later, she had bronchitis and pneumonia at the same time and was treated with both amoxicillin and Erythromycin. She added that she has had a lot of stress in her life, including having had several businesses fail, having been divorced, and having had the bank repossess her house.

Natalie   In 1978 Natalie had swollen glands in her neck from a cat scratch, and she took Keflex for a week. "After that I felt ill and started noticing strange pains," she said. Her symptoms continued even after physicians removed the glands in her neck. "Maybe my lymphatic system was disrupted. I still have problems in that area." She also drank a great deal of fruit juices. "I wasn't ever big on sweets, but I did have a lot of grape and apple juice," she said.

Pauline   About three months before she married at age eighteen, Pauline went on birth control pills, which she continued until she realized they were causing her health problems. When she first went on the pill, she had adverse reactions, including weight gain, elevated blood pressure, and increased premenstrual syndrome problems. She also had two or three bouts with vaginal yeast infections. In the first three months, she gained fifteen pounds, and the migraine headaches she'd had as a teenager started again. She also had mood swings and was always tired. She said taking birth control pills completely changed her health for the worse. Pauline said she also used to be addicted to sugar, which no doubt influenced her CRC.

Roger   Roger said the stress and grief of being divorced after ten years of marriage actually triggered his CRC, although his history of antibiotics and prednisone certainly contributed by depressing his immune system. "Within two or three years, I was very sick. I ran myself into the ground in my mid-thirties. I probably had it my whole life and just really had to face it nine years ago." Although he had some symptoms and health problems prior to the divorce, his health became much worse at that time. He became so weak he could barely walk across the room. "I needed bed rest to survive."

Roger thinks one cause of Candida is codependency. He also thinks Candida is brought on when people try to do too much and put more stress on themselves than their bodies can handle. He compared the CRC personality to the multiple sclerosis personality and said, "If the MS personality just backs off, they get better. The same applies to the CRC personality. People put so much on the body that the body can't take it."

Roger said that throughout his life he has been both ill and well at the same time. He described himself as having an iron will; he never let his general unwellness stop him from pursuing athletics and having a full life. "I probably pushed myself beyond my limits."

This is an important question because it goes beyond the technical aspects of CRC and helps us peek into the daily lives of each person. As in many of the responses to the following questions, the overall replies are similar, but each person adds something unique to the total answer.

What were the reactions of your friends, family, and coworkers to your health problems?

Blair   Blair's mysterious and unresolvable health problems led to marital problems with her husband. Blair said her husband thought she was crazy and that she and her husband would fight specifically about the length of her illness and about her medical bills. She said her health would further deteriorate after such domestic squabbles.

Blair added that part of the problem was that when she started feeling better, she would try to prove it to her husband and would consequently overextend herself and make her health worse. After she overdid herself, it would then take her several weeks to recoup her strength.

Beverly   "My family was sympathetic and supportive," said Beverly. "My coworkers were also, and [they were] concerned when I came down with hepatitis of an unknown origin. My family urged me to quit my job because I had never been so sick in all my life, but at the time I had no reason to think that I could get sick from working in a hospital. As I was to find out later, I was very wrong."

Dora   Dora said her health problems were extremely hard on her. When she became sick in 1989 people were less aware and less understanding of environmental sensitivities, although her husband supported her. "You find out who your friends are and those that will stick with you and do all the extras," she said.

One way Dora tried to reduce her exposure to chemicals was by putting a sign on her front door asking people not to wear after-shave inside her house. As a result, fewer people came to her house. She said she had a brother-in-law who would wear sweaters to her house that had been stored in mothballs, and it would make her extremely sick. "It was really hard to get across to people how I felt." The reactions of her friends and family to her environmental sensitivities led her to believe they considered themselves and the chemicals they wore to her house to be exceptions to her problems. "Some people refuse to believe you and think you mean everyone but them."

Deborah   Deborah didn't have much support from the people around her. "I'm sure lots of people thought I was not as troubled as I really was. The one doctor that I had for eighteen years said to me, 'There is nothing wrong with you.' "

Johanna   Johanna reported having both support and disbelief directed her way. "It's one of those things where just because your arm isn't falling off or you don't have big scabs on your face, people don't see how you can be sick." Johanna told of one skeptical relative who, not meaning to be insensitive, said, "But you don't look sick!"

Johanna said her husband has always been supportive, and her coworkers were both understanding and sorry she was sick.

She isn't close to her family and doesn't really have any close friends. "My family is basically disinterested, which is painful for me. I really don't have any support from family or friends about anything."

Kristy

"I tried to hide it for a long time, but I kept getting worse," said Kristy. "I tried to keep doing what I was doing. I wanted to take care of everyone else; I had to take care of everyone else. I was into the mentality of taking care of everyone, but no one could take care of me." Finally she became too sick to keep up a pretense of being well and had to explain to her three children about her health problems. "It was very difficult," she said.

But Kristy added that her illness had an beneficial effect on her family. "My family is much healthier because of my illness. My family was very supportive. This has been a strengthening experience for all of us and has made us much closer. For a lifetime, we're all the better for it."

Marla

Marla said at first her family had trouble believing yeast could cause overall health problems, but they gradually became aware there was more to CRC than just yeast. She said her health problems affected the entire family. Her condition influenced what they ate and whether or not they used antibiotics, especially in relation to the grandchildren. "Everybody started to see there was something to it."

She described her husband as being tolerant of her health problems. "My husband [who had congenitive heart failure] has really learned what a difference it makes to watch his diet." Her husband, who had problems with depression and digestion, found that changing his diet and taking acidophilus several times a day helped him a great deal. "His attitude was much better," she added.

Megan

"My family was super, but it took a toll on them," said Megan. Her illness first occurred when she became engaged to her present husband. "I was so sick it was hard to be romantic."

Other people were not as understanding as her family. "I never heard anyone say I was crazy, but I felt it from people. Well, I did hear it from doctors." She said she would go out of her way to avoid mentioning her illness to anyone. "I always felt odd describing it to people. I know people thought I was taking this too far. The problem is this mostly affects women, and their word is not important."

Mary Jo

Mary Jo said the people around her, her friends and family, were understanding of her health problems. "They thought the diet was nuts, though. It made perfect sense to me."

Natalie   Natalie said because she lives far from her family, no one knew about her health problems. "I didn't complain to anyone, so no one knew my suffering."

Pauline   "Some of my friends have the same problems," said Pauline. While her husband is supportive of her, she reported that some of her friends are not so lucky. She has one friend whose husband supports her only to a certain degree, and she has other friends with husbands who provide financial but not psychological support.

"Others don't understand it. People tend to dismiss them [my health problems] as laziness. I've learned to keep them to myself as a form of protection. They really don't understand it. It got to the point where I didn't need support—or I guess I needed it, but knew I wouldn't get it. I think people would be much better if they had support from their families. It's really a shame."

Roger   Roger said he felt isolated and was criticized by the people around him. "People said I looked fine." He was highly criticized by his coworkers: "People think you're weird. It's a definite disability." He observed that when people don't feel well, they tend to become introverted, which can attract even more criticism.

What is the best first step to take? Many of these thirteen patients ended up doing one of two things: they began working with a physician toward treating their illness or they started by treating themselves and at the same time searched for a physician who treated CRC. When speaking of their search for doctors, many were hopeful and resigned at the same time. Ironically, the two feelings do go together. Many realized doctors were key to their recovery, and yet they'd been disappointed by so many doctors that they knew the task of finding the doctor to fit their needs would not be an easy one.

What did you do first? Did you have trouble finding a doctor?

Blair   After treating herself for three months, Blair found a chiropractor with a treatment plan that included blood-purifying agents, acidophilus, adding fiber to the diet, and following the anti-Candida diet. She found a physician in a neighboring state and followed her program for about six months, but she still had some problems because she didn't strictly follow the prescribed anti-Candida diet. "It helped, but I still wanted to have sugar. I didn't get totally well, but I did improve." She said the reason she didn't get well was because she had been trying to fool her system and had been eating sugar substitutes and other prohibited foods.

Beverly   "I had trouble finding a doctor that would listen to me, but I kept going until I found a doctor who knew what I was going through," said Beverly.

Dora   After a physician suggested Candida might be her problem, Dora, an avid reader, immediately read more about Candida and realized it was causing her illness.

Deborah   Deborah said she stayed with the nutritionist and also started going to a reflexologist. "They both helped me. But I still studied all the literature and books that I could find on the treatment for Candida. I also dealt with a M.D. in Arizona who did not use medicine. He treats nutritional and stress-related problems. He is very good. He did hair analysis, which is an excellent way of finding out your body nutrients and what is out of balance."

Megan   Even after Megan managed to get a diagnosis and searched for a doctor to help her, she said, "I couldn't find anyone who would lend it any credence. Many more doctors are now giving it credence. They are starting to listen to their patients, but still if I had a problem, I wouldn't go to them."

Marla   Marla first visited a female physician who had been recommended to her and who she described as being sympathetic to the idea. "Male doctors are so hard to convince," she added. Her blood test showed an abnormally high count of Candida, and the physician prescribed nystatin. However, she reported that her present physician, who happens to be male, works with her and listens better than many other doctors she has spoken to.

Natalie   Natalie immediately went out and bought a book and started the diet. "The book made a lot of sense." Since she couldn't find a doctor, she basically treated her CRC herself.

Pauline   One of Pauline's friends had gone to a physician in Memphis, and Pauline went to him also. She filled out a questionnaire and had some blood tests done, which confirmed she had CRC.

Roger   Like many patients, Roger went from one doctor to another trying to discover answers. Since he didn't have any success, he turned to books and started finding solutions. He did get some help from the physician who diagnosed his CRC and CFS, however.

A surprising amount of people don't go to doctors at all and are able to take care of their own problems, though others visit physicians who practice a variety of medical techniques and theories.

What kind of doctor are you going to about your Candida-related problems?

Beverly	Beverly is going to both an environmental doctor and a family doctor. "The family doctor does not accept the treatment that is given by my other doctor. This is too bad because I know the need for these doctors to spend some time on this problem," she said.
Deborah	"I am now going to a D.O. who treats Candida—he also does chelation therapy," reported Deborah. "He runs a preventative health care clinic and is very good. He feels that about 90 percent of people walking around have Candida to some extent, and I agree."
Kristy	When Kristy first became ill, she had difficulty discovering what she had. "It was very hard to find a doctor who realized what my problems were," Kristy said. Doctors would try to give her nerve pills or antidepressant drugs, and none really helped her. "I knew there was nothing wrong mentally."
	She said that now when she goes to a new doctor she "interviews" him to find out whether or not he's what she wants. If the physician objects to her questions, she gets up and leaves because she knows he is not the type of physician she needs. "I have had the most help from the doctors least concerned with making money."
Megan	Like many CRC patients, Megan takes care of her own health problems. "I don't go to doctors. I do it all myself, and I don't get sick." She is pregnant with her third child and delivered her second child at home with the help of an obstetrician. The physician, an eighty-seven-year-old woman who works full-time, will also assist in the delivery of her third child.
	No one in Megan's immediate family ever seems to get sick, even the children. "Fifty percent of illness is a state of mind. Not all of it—this isn't in people's heads. We use a lot of spirituality to heal ourselves—and it works. We also do a lot of praying for our health," she said.
Natalie	"I don't go to doctors; I don't have any faith in them," said Natalie. "I would rather cure myself than go to a doctor. That would change if I found one who was more nutritionally oriented."

Pauline   Because she just moved, Pauline is in between doctors and currently going to two chiropractors. She said they understand how Candida works and how the supplements she takes work. She goes to them for guidance and also goes to her gynecologist for her yearly checkup. "I keep myself up so there are no emergencies," she said. She would like to find a doctor who practices alternative medicine to go to for guidance, for general health problems, and for times when there are serious problems. "I know my knowledge is limited."

Pauline commented on how doctors respond, without even realizing it, to the expectations of their patients. She told about her experiences with one physician whom she refused to let dictate to her. She instead demanded they discuss her problems. "He respected me for that, for being prepared, for thinking about the choices he presented, and for not just being willing to walk out the door with a handful of drugs."

Roger   "I haven't been to a doctor in a long time," said Roger. "I don't need them anymore. Anything that hits me, I can treat myself. I know that sounds crazy, but it works." Roger hasn't been to a doctor in four years, but if he needed to go he would. "I go by how I feel and how my body is functioning."

Treatments varied from the standard medications prescribed by physicians to remedies found in health food stores.

What treatments have you tried? What did your doctor recommend?

Blair   Blair felt worse after starting the treatment, much worse than the symptoms which had been explained to her. "I think I was trying to kill it off too fast—I just wanted it to be gone," she said.

She successfully treated her eczema using three to four Taheebo tea capsules a day. She also had colonics and did chelation therapy. Another treatment that really helped her vaginal infections was topical treatment of her vaginal canal with garlic and nystatin, which she did under the supervision of a physician.

Beverly   Beverly found natural products helpful. "I was put on antifungal medicine and an individualized program of vitamins, minerals, food concentrates, digestive enzymes, and raw glandulars. All the products are yeast-free and self-tested for sensitivity reactions. Now I avoid antibiotics, immunosuppressant drugs and oral contraceptives. I also avoid foods known to feed Candida," she said.

Deborah   "The D.O. had me use many vitamins and mineral supplements plus nystatin, and the nystatin he uses is from Canada and is pure," said Deborah. "What is prescribed here in the States has coloring added, which is not good.

"I was checked for food allergies, and I had twenty-two, so I went three months without all twenty-two foods. Now I rotate my foods and seem to get along pretty well. I'm sure I will always have to be very careful with my diet because the Candida can flare up very easily. I also use acidophilus and glandular products to help build up my immune system, and I use thymus, pituitary, and adrenal glandulars. I also use herbs. I do not use nystatin anymore; I use caprylic acid," she said.

Jonathon   Jonathon's allergist put him on a very restrictive yeast- and sugar-free diet and gave him allergy shots. Before seeing this doctor, he had made some progress with steroid therapy. "The treatment for this problem is not a quick fix. Like all health care, you manage it."

Johanna   Johanna is currently seeing a doctor in Ohio, two hours away from her home, and so far she has visited him three times. "I'm pleased for the most part with him, but he doesn't always take the time to explain things," she said. She finds this very frustrating.

Her doctor recommended the diet and gave her a prescription for Diflucan. Johanna said she is unhappy about the diet. "It's confusing. The information is conflicting because people are still finding out about it. What exactly can I eat?" She added that although sugar is an obvious and clear-cut example of what to avoid, she is confused about what other foods she can and cannot eat. "I feel from time to time that I'm winging it from day to day. I put stuff in my mouth and hope it's the right thing."

Kristy   Kristy did take nystatin, but was uncertain whether it helped her. "I never could tell if it made a difference for me." She thinks it may have helped in conjunction with the colonic irrigation. "If I had colonics while taking the nystatin I would have felt much better."

She doesn't want to take drugs and would explain to her physicians that using medications wasn't the route she wanted to take. "I decided a long time ago I would not participate in these medications. As long as I'm making progress, I won't take drugs."

Because of her gastrointestinal problems, she has been very careful about what she eats. When she tested herself for food allergies through an elimination diet, she was able to pinpoint the foods she was allergic to. Although she did strictly follow the diet for a year and a half, she didn't think that really helped her health as much as using the remedies available at health food stores.

Marla　Marla found nystatin very helpful. She did try the yeast-fighting medications from the health food store, but didn't find them very helpful. "They may help when the problem is light, but I wouldn't think they would touch the serious stuff. They work too slowly." She said the nystatin helped her very much.

Megan　Megan was on nystatin for about eight months, but she regrets taking it. "That was a mistake; I don't think I should have taken that. As soon as you start with 'let's kill it' instead of 'let's build the immune system,' you're in trouble."

She also took vitamins to restore the lost nutrients in her body. "Looking back, a better route would have been vitamin-packed foods. It was the right direction at least." Megan said what helped the most, however, was cutting out white flour, coffee, white sugar, and anything processed. She also avoids alcohol. Megan also tried *Lactobacillus acidophilus* but said it was hard to know exactly what really helped. "It certainly contributed," she said.

Mary Jo　"I felt incredibly fragile, as if the slightest thing would set me off," said Mary Jo. After moving, she found a physician who was both an M.D. and a kinesiologist, and she said he continues to help her tremendously. The doctor prescribed Nizerol and nystatin, and she found that the nystatin helped a great deal.

Natalie　After a friend told her about CRC, Natalie went on the anti-Candida diet. "The diet was depressing," she remembered. She also took acidophilus and a nonprescription anti-Candida medication called yeast-fighters, which she said really helped. She also had her mercury amalgam fillings removed and immediately felt better.

Pauline　Pauline's doctor put her on nystatin, but she said her stomach couldn't handle it. In retrospect, she thinks her adverse reactions may have been just the die-off symptoms. Pauline said when it comes to treating her CRC she has been lucky: "Through the years the things I do always seem to help."

Roger   Roger's physician gave him nystatin, Nizerol, and amphotericin B. "They didn't help, and they may have hurt me. They also suppress the immune system." In addition he had severe symptoms from the Candida die-off: "The die-off was so bad I was hallucinating."

Roger decided to heal himself naturally and used garlic, the Candida control diet, and the over-the-counter antifungal medications available at health food stores. "The diet helped for a while, but I started to feel bad again. I realized I needed to do more than the doctor could do for me," he said. He also exercised by walking at a brisk pace and took deep breaths, being careful to fully exhale all the air from his lungs.

Although this question had to be phrased neutrally, most everyone found the implication that CRC did not change their life to be at the least surprising and at the most a little offensive.

Has this illness changed your life? If so, how?

Blair   "It's all but destroyed it!" Blair laughed. "When you don't feel like yourself, it affects you and your family." She described herself as a "semifunctioning vegetable" and said, "I could always do some things. I always managed to take care of the kids."

Beverly   "Yes, this has changed my life," said Beverly. "I had to take an early retirement because I developed a lot of allergies to foods and chemicals. Now I can't wear makeup or perfume. I do not eat out much because of all the food allergies I have."

Dora   Even though she feels much better, Dora is still severely restricted by her adverse reactions to personal-care products. Because of this, she doesn't know if she can ever work or be around other people again. "It's too hard to be around people who won't work with me," she said. As a result of her chemical sensitivities, she has to stay in the house permanently and limit her activities: "I feel like I'm in a cage because I like to cook and eat the food I cook." Whenever possible, she said, she tries to educate people about environmental illness and Candida.

Deborah   Deborah reported she was feeling much better. "I am in much better health now but I still need help, so I am hoping the removal of the amalgam fillings [which are over 50 percent mercury] will be of help."

Jonathon   "This changed the whole focus of my professional and personal life," said Jonathon. "I had to give up my house because it was so infested with mold." He was also forced to relocate to a drier climate. Because of his health problems, he couldn't get a job, so he opened a business that is almost unique: a pharmacy/ health food store.

Johanna   Johanna is having difficulty adjusting to the changes in her life. She mentioned her inability to tolerate inks, which keeps her from reading, and the fact that she can no longer eat fruit, which she dearly loves. She finds not being able to read especially frustrating. "I walk around frustrated all the time, hoping I'll get better."

Kristy   Like many people who have experienced CRC, Kristy offered clear insights on how Candida thoroughly changed her life. "Yes [this has changed my life]. It made me patient with other people and patient with myself. I'm a better person because of this. I was always very intolerant of other people's weaknesses." She said she realizes the importance of stopping and resting when necessary and having patience with her health. "Now it's part of my day to take care of myself. I now plan out what food I'm going to eat." She said she's slowed down a lot and hired people to come to her house and do projects she previously would have tried to do herself.

"I've gone through a lot of feelings, emotions because of this," she said. Kristy learned a great deal about herself. "I found my body could only do so much. Sooner or later, we all pay for it." She added, "I can't take care of anyone else if I don't take care of myself.

"Time is very precious," she continued. "Learn to value what's really important. When my teenagers talk to me now, I stop what I'm doing, look right at them, and listen to every word they say. I try to make my time count. I don't mind being different. If I have different needs, it's worth it to me to take care of them. I don't follow the crowd."

Megan   Megan said her illness has made her a better mother, and if she had had her children at a younger age, her relationship with them would have been very different. "Motherhood is my joy, my nourishment. I am appreciative of being a mother and completely enjoy motherhood."

Megan describes the effect CRC had on her as cleansing and says the overall result was beneficial because it helped her grow and mature. "I'm a completely different person," she said. "I think I'm more careful, patient, and less aggressive. I look at this illness as a blessing despite the toll it took on me. And it gave me insight into life and an appreciation of life that's incredible." She said her illness added spirituality to her life. "It gave me religion; before I never even believed in God. I didn't find religion until the end, and that's what clinched my health. That was definitely a very large force in curing me.

"It changed me in every possible way," she continued. "Then I was a Republican, and now I'm as far left as I can be. My goals used to be material and getting ahead socially and professionally. Now my goals are to care for my family and get in touch with the really important issues—the issues of being human."

Mary Jo   Mary Jo said her health problems have helped her to a certain extent. She said, at first she was very upset and would cry every night, but because of her CRC, she started going to church again. She also reduced the pressure she puts on herself. "I've stopped doing anything strenuous or stressful," she said.

Natalie   Natalie said having CRC has helped her improve her diet: "I try to eat better."

She also said she realized the importance of taking care of herself. "I realized how special our body machinery is. You don't have time to indulge and put junk in your body. We have the opportunity to do things that are good for us," she said.

Pauline   Pauline said CRC has changed her life and the way she looks at her health. "There are times when I wish I didn't know all this—it's so much trouble. But it has saved me a lot of pain and helped a lot." She described herself as being open-minded because of her health problems. "Overall I feel less trusting, but at the same time more open-minded than other people. I can see both sides." She is also grateful she has taken a natural approach to healing herself: "I can't imagine where we [my family] would be if I took traditional medical treatments like drugs or surgery."

Roger   "Oh, yes. I'm learning to say no instead of allowing myself to be sucked dry. I feel so much more at peace." Roger said he has learned to respect himself, and because of his CRC, he has gotten to know who he really is: "I do everything in the extreme. I think that's a common thread among CRC and CFS people." Roger said that throughout his life he has been constantly plagued with doubts and felt lost and on his own. As a codependent personality, he latched onto relationships as a way to avoid looking inside himself and facing painful truths. He added that five years of attending a support group for codependency helped him get his life back on track. "The codependen-cy therapy probably saved my life," he said. Through the thera-py, he learned how to stop "caretaking" others and how to set limits. "It's all about not controlling or being controlled." He concluded: "My Candida did me one big favor."

Thankfully only a few of the respondents' children had Candida-related problems. Many of the men and women did not have children or did not mention them in relation to having health problems with Candida.

Has your children's health been affected by Candida?

Blair   Two of Blair's children were started on antibiotics immediately after being born, and the other was also started at a young age. All had various infections, including sinus, tonsil, and ear infections. Her problems with Candida were passed to both her daughters at birth, and both had thrush, though her son did not since he was born by C-section and therefore didn't pass through the birth canal. All three children have been healthy since she stopped giving them antibiotics three years ago. Instead of using antibiotics, she has been treating their minor ailments with herbs.

Since she takes care of other children besides her own, she has had a chance to talk to other mothers of young children and said some children are given antibiotics for problems as simple as a runny nose. "They [doctors] are practicing too much preventative medicine," she added. As another example of excessive preventative medicine, Blair said, before she stopped giving her children antibiotics one physician told her he was going to put her daughter, who was sick with the flu, on an antibiotic because there was a 15 percent chance she would develop an ear infection after recovering from the flu.

Jonathon   Jonathon said the only problems his children have are allergies.

Marla   Marla said one of her daughters and one of her sons, both of whom had antibiotics as children, have had problems with Candida. She added that in retrospect she thinks their depres-sion during their teen years may have been tied to Candida. She said her son has both extreme sweets cravings and a diet high in sugar. He also has problems with depression. Marla reported her daughter had a lot of trouble getting pregnant, but after she went on the Candida control diet she was able to get pregnant.

Megan   Thankfully Megan's children haven't had any Candida-related problems. "Maybe once a year they have a cold. We never have to worry about it. They just don't get sick." Other than an ear infection her son, who is now seven years old, had when he was two, her children are perfectly healthy and have never had aspirin, Tylenol, or antibiotics.

She said that she and her husband have taught their children that sickness isn't something they should be afraid of. "They don't look at it as a fearful thing. We tell them they are protected and cared for by God no matter what ache they have. If we look at ourselves as material, that's what we'll expect. If we look at ourselves as spiritual, that's what we'll expect."

Pauline   Pauline said her oldest son, who is now sixteen years old, also had trouble with Candida. When he was young, he had immune system problems that stemmed from Candida. Through a careful diet they were able to get his immune problems under control. She said that early on in his life he hadn't been exposed to much stress, but when he began to go through puberty, the amount of stress in his life increased and his Candida problems resumed. "We had some years where things were under control," added Pauline. But, when puberty began, "we were caught off guard." Around puberty he began to have skin rashes, allergies, and to gain weight.

While everyone found different methods and approaches helpful, the most frequently mentioned treatments include vitamins, acidophilus, the Candida control diet, and prescription medications.

What helped you the most?

Blair   Blair said the colonics, her strict Candida control diet, nystatin, and the chelation therapy have helped her the most. She added that in trying to recover from CRC, she has accumulated about $30,000 to $35,000 of debt on her credit cards from the various doctors and medications she has tried. "When I would read about stuff in the books, I would immediately go and try it whatever the price," she said. At one point she was taking seventy-five pills a day, mostly vitamins and supplements, which she said did help tremendously.

Beverly   "What has helped me most was to finally find out what was wrong with me and to know what to do about it," said Beverly.

Dora   "I was fortunate because I had discipline," said Dora. "Now I don't have any patience with people who aren't disciplined." Dora found several ways to help herself feel better. One thing that greatly helped was making her house her sanctuary, which she accomplished by throwing out everything that made her ill, including all chemical products, perfumes, and wall-to-wall carpets. Even years later, she said she would continue to find items around her house that would make her sick. Another way she avoided chemicals was to avoid using commercial cleansing products. Dora said she uses what her grandmother used to clean around the house: baking soda and other natural cleaners. "It's amazing—you really don't need all those individual cleaners."

Another big help was going to a sauna because sweating is a natural way of excreting toxins from the body. "I swear that's what made me better," she declared. In an effort to avoid people (because of their scented products), she went early in the morning. Taking garlic pills every day also helped, as did introducing new foods from time to time to see how they affected her. "You have to find out for yourself what you can and can't eat. Everyone is different."

Deborah   "My positive attitude tells me I can get better and that there is help. I just keep looking for it," said Deborah. "Do not settle for the 'there is nothing more I can do' attitude of so many doctors."

Johanna   "As far as I can tell," said Johanna, "the Diflucan and the diet in conjunction. I have the added difficulty of not knowing if I'm getting better because of the Chronic Fatigue Syndrome. I need to get the Candida under control before we work on the Chronic Fatigue."

Kristy   Kristy said acidophilus, aloe vera juice, and chlorophyll (which is good for intestinal problems) really helped her get better. She has also found it crucial to not only eat the foods right for her, but to also do "proper food combining" and eat certain foods at certain times of the day. "I feel like I've been on the right track."

Kristy has visited several different types of alternative physicians, including herbalists, acupressurists, and reflexologists. "I went without expectations of a miracle, and I learned something from each one of them. Everyone played a role." One method she found extremely helpful was contact reflex analysis (CRA). This method finds the points of the body that are weak and is similar to kinesiology, which is the study of muscular activity in the body. "I would definitely vouch for that," she said.

Marla   Marla said the nystatin and acidophilus have helped her the most. "Nystatin is by far the fastest." She has also found that staying away from sweets, starchy foods, and milk really helps. "I feel a lot better when I don't have milk." For her skin problems, she has found Nizerol creams help reduce scaling and itching.

Megan   Megan said what helped her the most was the spirituality she developed as a result of the illness. "That transcends every- thing," she said. What also helped was changing her diet to include organically grown foods and using herbs to cure her- self. She also found homeopathy helped a great deal.

Natalie   Natalie found changing her diet helpful: "After I changed my diet, I felt really good." She added, "I used to notice this before I went on the diet: I would eat junk in December and would feel bad, mainly aches and pains, in January and February." She also found acidophilus beneficial.

Pauline   Pauline said, after she realized what the problem was, she did a lot of reading and research on Candida. Two things she learned that have helped her are that fiber and aloe vera juice help alle- viate constipation and other digestive problems.

"I have some basic things I fall back on that have been good for me." She said two things that help her are vitamin supplements and keeping the toxins produced by Candida out of her body by keeping her kidneys and colon cleansed through vitamin/mineral supplements. The number one supplement Pauline recommended was digestive enzymes, which can be purchased at health food stores. She said that within thirty minutes of taking digestive enzymes her symptoms would be gone. "Everything starts with digestion. You can't get the nutri- ents you need if your digestion isn't working properly." The enzymes are needed because the body is so taxed it can't pro- duce its own enzymes. The added enzymes help support the organs; this not only aids digestion but also helps take stress off the body.

Pauline also found that writing about her health and symp- toms helped her and gave her perspective on her health prob- lems. "Keeping a journal helped me see the connections between circumstances around me and my health problems." For example, she discovered that her arguments with her hus- band coincided with her menstrual periods.

Roger   Roger said what helped him the most was using a total approach, which he described as including herbs, homeopathic medicine, a diet of raw foods, and trying not to internalize stress. He also cut caffeine, alcohol, stimulants, red meat, and chicken out of his diet. "To be healthy is so simple. Eat healthy, get rest, think positively, be happy, and exercise. Do that, and you'll be OK. It seems so basic, yet people ignore it."

He also makes sure he gets the vitamins and minerals he needs and eats a high-fiber diet. He uses coffee enemas to help rebuild his liver cells. They also help get rid of a lot of body waste and clean out the colon," he said. For Roger, working on problems one at a time and working toward a balanced life helped him improve his health. He also had his mercury amalgams removed. "Let me tell you—the amount of mercury in one filling is enough to kill you," he claimed.

He has also found that drinking organically grown and freshly pressed apple and carrot juice is very helpful. "When you use organically grown vegetables you get the minerals you need." He also recommended drinking a mixture of puréed green leafy vegetables called a "green drink." He stresses that to get the maximum amount of vitamins and minerals out of foods, they need to be eaten raw: "Don't cook food over 120 degrees or it's dead; there are no vitamins and minerals left."

Roger said everything he has found helpful came as the result of reading and dredging through a lot of books. "I believe in the eclectic approach; do what works and what doesn't hurt the body," he said. But most importantly, he said the best approach is to reduce activity and stress. "If I don't feel well, all I have to do is calm down, slow down, and do everything right."

Suggestions ranged from which approaches to take to CRC, to advice on what to do and what not to do, to reassurances that complete recovery is possible.

What advice would you give someone with Candida-related problems? What do you recommend?

Blair   Blair suggested that, depending the situation of each patient, colonics might help. Otherwise she recommended acidophilus, Taheebo tea, the Candida control diet, and a good multiple vitamin with extra B-complex. "Before they start all that, they really need to get their colon cleaned out," she adds. "If the [toxic products from] die-off can't move out of the system, you're going to get sick, really sick."

Beverly   Beverly said she would recommend that patients stick to the Candida control diet as closely as possible, join a support group if one is near, and try to learn as much as they can. "They should also talk to their doctors about what they have learned. These doctors need to be educated about this problem."

Dora

Dora cheerfully offered inspirational advice on the inevitability of getting better: "Hang in there and do what you have to do. Getting well is very hard and difficult, but it will happen." She emphasized the importance of following the Candida control diet as well. "The diet is very important. If you cheat, you'll pay for it."

She also offered advice on dealing with doctors who treat CRC. "I think there are probably some charlatans making some money from it," she said. She also has a problem with some of the symptoms tests administered by physicians who treat Candida. "Some tests are so vague they could apply to anyone. Be careful not to fall in a trap."

Deborah

Deborah also offered encouraging advice. "Find a nutritionally oriented doctor that really believes in Candida. They do exist," she said.

Jonathon

Jonathon said he informally advises about one hundred men, women, and children about their Candida-related problems. "I let them know number one is the diet. I also let them know the anti-Candida drugs that are available, both prescription and nonprescription."

Many of the people who come in to his pharmacy/health food store have food sensitivities and food allergies. Others are aware they have Candida-related problems but aren't ready to make the necessary lifestyle changes. "I get people in here who know what the problem is but won't do the diet."

Three nonprescription methods available are caprylic acid, which he said works on some people and seems to help women with vaginitis. Two other popular methods are echinacea and acidophilus. Jonathon said he sells a lot of acidophilus and has a whole bottom refrigerator shelf of different types of nystatin. "Just in this little backwater area I have dozens of bottles of nystatin." He also sells a daily tea for Candida he makes himself of Pau d'arco, echinacea, lemon grass, peppermint, hibiscus flowers, rose hips, cinnamon, licorice root, and stevia.

He recommended that when patients are feeling better they should challenge themselves with suspicious foods. And he recommended patients take acidophilus whenever they have to take antibiotics. "Anytime I give a prescription for antibiotics I tell them to have yogurt—real yogurt, not that Dannon syrupy stuff."

Johanna

Johanna emphasized the importance of patients educating themselves. "Providing they can read books, I would recommend they read everything they can get their hands on. They might also want to find a support group. The irony, of course, is that if you're sick you can't do stuff like that easily."

Kristy   "To me, the most important thing is attitude," said Kristy. "At first I thought, why me? I felt like a victim. Why do I have to be sick at the most important time in my life, which is when my children are young? I felt guilty for not being able to take care of them. I felt guilty because my husband had to do so much." She learned to put aside her guilt and feelings of inadequacy, although she said it was hard to accept at first. "I'm worthy of the extra attention I need right now. I'm worthy of getting well, and I expect that to happen."

Kristy highly recommended colonic irrigation. Kristy described the process as being similar to any other that involves simple cleansing with water. She added that for her, colonic irrigation was "a lot more than an enema." The actual process involves passing a rubber tube about twenty to thirty inches into the rectum. Several gallons of warm water are then pumped in and out, and various substances from the body come out in the water.

Kristy said she found colonic irrigation to be extremely helpful. She had twelve treatments over several months, with a treatment about every two weeks. About the process she said: "I felt great twelve times over." She and a friend drove six hours each way to the natural health clinic in the next state that performed colonic irrigations. They would have a colonic when they arrived, stay overnight in a hotel, and have another colonic before they drove back the next day. "I've traveled to get the help I needed." She said that at the price of about $80, a treatment was well worth it. "I've paid a lot more for things that didn't help. It's not expensive if it helps." She recommended colonic irrigation to anyone who needs to get Candida overgrowth out of their large intestine.

Describing how she felt between the colonic irrigation sessions, she said, "I just kept getting better and better. By the time I finished, I was a totally new person." She described her improvement as around 50 percent. For more information on colonic irrigation see the chapter on additional treatments for CRC.

Marla   Marla offered both supportive and inspirational advice. She recommended that people straighten out their diet and also said that "to lie around and feel sorry for yourself drags it out." She emphasized the importance of finding a good doctor. "It's important for your morale to have someone who works with you. Seek out a doctor who will use a thorough treatment. Don't go to a doctor who drags the treatment out."

Megan   Megan offered both encouragement and support. "I was really sick for a long time, and I know it's possible to cure this; I feel very strongly about it. If I can do it, other people can do it. It's not just me. I know others that have been cured, too."

She also urged patients to take full responsibility for their health. "It's up to you to ask questions, do your own research, and then make the decisions." She added that recovering from CRC takes patience. "It takes a lot of time, and that's an important thing to remember. Everyone has their own path. If you look you will find it. After you get rid of your angry emotions [about being ill], your intuition will surface. Follow that; it will just come to you."

Mary Jo   Mary Jo offered three suggestions. She emphasized the importance of diet: "They've got to change their food habits, and it's the hardest thing to do." She also recommended the place where she was able to find the help she needed. She said, "Go to health food stores. The information is there that you can't find anywhere else." And finally, she stressed the need to find a physician who is familiar with CRC.

Natalie   Natalie offered two helpful hints. The first is to "watch fruit juices." She also recommended acidophilus, which she said still helps her now: "Candida or not, taking the acidophilus makes me feel better, gives me more strength."

Pauline   Pauline spoke with a mixture of caution and optimism, and most of her advice concerned how to best work with physicians. About doctors she said, "You don't have to do exactly what they say. I try to get people to think about what options are out there. If they're not ready for it, they're not going to do it anyway." She said many people think that doctors know everything, so they don't think to look at the alternatives which may be available. "Because of that there is a lot of needless pain."

She urges patients not to let doctors have too much control over their lives. "Don't take an M.D.'s word as law. There is plenty of research out there on your problems. There is so much we can all do. People could do more for themselves if they tried; take control of your health." She emphasized the need to have faith and trust in yourself: "Don't give up because your M.D. says there is nothing wrong."

Roger   "I would tell them to immediately go on the diet and go on a raw food diet as much as possible," said Roger. "Go the natural route. I wouldn't take any medications. Medications just create more problems. You won't get well taking medications. You can get well if you treat yourself; no doctor will get you better. The only way a person can get well is to take charge of their health and use doctors as tools. No doctor I've met knows anywhere near what they need to know. Doctors treat it—they don't get you over it."

Roger also emphasized the basics: getting enough aerobic exercise, eating correctly, and getting enough sleep and relaxation. "If you don't get your rest, you don't stand a chance of recovering." He also added, "It [CRC] is complex, but it's also simple if people understand the basics. So many people say 'Why me?' and I say to them 'Why not you?' Look at your habits."

He recommended the use of remedies available at health food stores, such as flaxseed oil, which builds up the essential fatty acids (EFAs) necessary for health, and Ginkgo biloba, which boosts mental clarity by helping blood get to the brain. He also stressed the importance of getting personal affairs in order. "Check out the possibility of codependency and the spiritual side of life."

Lifestyle changes among the patients ranged from more care taken concerning food and eating to different attitudes toward life and living. Everyone interpreted this question a little differently, providing a broad range of responses.

Do you do things now that you didn't do before? Has your lifestyle stayed the same or changed?

Beverly   "Well, I now eat more health foods than I used to and cook more veggies," said Beverly. "I also have become more careful of the environment. I am always telling people about how important it is to read the labels at the grocery store; it would shock them to see some of the stuff they are putting in their bodies."

Dora   Dora said the hardest thing was giving up her social life. Even though she feels a lot better, she said she continues to avoid crowds and to not eat out a lot. However, the no-smoking policy many restaurants have adopted could make dining out a little easier, she said.

Deborah   Deborah said her lifestyle is about the same, but because of her age she has slowed down.

Jonathon   Jonathon said his lifestyle has changed quite a bit. He said, "I never eat out. Hardly, hardly ever. I only eat stuff I have here [in the health food store] and organic produce." He said he never eats sugar or red meat. "I haven't had red meat in years, not because I have anything against meat, but because I can't stand the antibiotics and steroids. I have plenty of available protein sources without it."

Because of his health problems, he realized diet has a great deal to do with illness. "Why do you think I have a health food store?" he asked.

Johanna   "It's pretty much stayed the same with the exception of not working," said Johanna. "And I can't go out to dinner because I can't eat anything on the menu." Since cleansing products and pine-scented products make her ill, she has also switched to natural cleaning products such as vinegar and baking soda.

Johanna also said some of her ideas about illness and doctors had changed. "The older and wiser I get, theoretically, I think I'm finding out what most people probably know already; you have to educate yourself in addition to going to a doctor," Johanna said. "I'm not implying doctors are ignorant, but there is so much out there that they can't know everything."

Kristy   Kristy used to measure her worth according to her accomplishments, but she no longer needs to do that. When she doesn't get all her work finished, she doesn't let it bother her. "I don't have to do all this today. Even though I didn't get everything I wanted to done, I can still value myself. Now I feel I should enjoy every day," she said. The guilt no longer torments her. She said she has realized "just because I'm sick doesn't make me any less of a person."

Currently she is continuing to work on stress reduction. "That's what I need to improve." She has also learned the importance of healing herself: "I have taken charge of my own health. It's not who can help me, but how I can better help myself. No one else can do for me what I can do for me. It's up to me to find what makes me well."

Kristy also said her family's lifestyles have changed. They eat better, take better care of their health, have more positive attitudes, and try not to let stress affect them so much. "Health is a blessing, not something you should take for granted."

Marla   "Over the years, I've become more interested in taking care of my health," said Marla. "I know how much good it does." She said she goes lightly on alcoholic drinks, having only an occasional cocktail or glass of wine. "That is the one thing that has changed the most in the last few years."

Megan   Megan said now she eats out from time to time, but before she recovered there were times she never would have gone to a restaurant. She said, "I just don't order things that are horrendous. Foods that are processed and loaded with chemicals just don't interest me anymore."

Megan has also drastically changed her eating habits and doesn't eat traditional food. She grinds her own flour and makes her own pasta, crackers, cheese, and bread. "When I don't, I don't buy it. It's my joy now. It represents more than keeping me healthy—it represents a lifestyle."

She also buys only organically grown fruits and vegetables, and she buys goat milk and eggs from people she trusts to not use chemicals or nonorganic methods. About five years ago she and a friend started a co-op. She said she did it because she had to find a way to get organic vegetables. During the winter, the co-op provides organically grown fruits and vegetables to the two hundred members in the area. In the summer, she takes her children to a local farm where food is grown organically to pick out their own produce. "It's fun and very exciting to do. I want my children to see what food is all about and that it doesn't grow in supermarkets."

Megan had to discontinue her community work because of her illness. She said that once she became sick, she couldn't go to meetings because of the perfumes everyone was wearing. "I had to bow out of everything."

Mary Jo   The changes in Mary Jo's life mainly revolve around her diet and food. "I eat virtually no dairy, and I haven't had meat in four years," she said. She explained that she doesn't eat meat because "your body doesn't digest it well, and psychologically I don't want to eat meat." She is also much more careful about what foods she buys. "I've become much more aware of food labels. I read everything."

Pauline   "I try to be informed about things," said Pauline. "I always knew my own mind, and in a lot of ways that's been a good thing."

Roger   Because of his health problems, Roger has developed an intense and lifelong interest in health, medicine, and CRC. "I spend my life thinking about this stuff because it fascinates me. A lot of people think I'm crazy to read so many health books."

RESOURCES

Suggested Readings

The following listings are intended as a first step toward identifying suitable resources for you and your family, not as recommendations of any program or medical professional.

Allergies

Allergy Cooking with Ease: The No Wheat, Milk, Eggs, Corn, Soy, Yeast, Sugar, Grain and Gluten Cookbook, by Nicolette M. Dumke (Starburst Publishers, 1992).

An Alternative Approach to Allergies, by Theron G. Randolph, M.D,. and R.W. Ross, Ph.D. (HarperCollins, 1990).

Brain Allergies: The Psychonutrient Connection, by William H. Philpot, M.D., and D. K. Kalita, Ph.D. (Keats Publishing, 1987).

The Complete Guide to Food Allergy and Intolerance, by Jonathan Brostoff and Linda Gammlin (Crown Publishing Group, 1992).

Detecting Your Hidden Allergies, by William G. Crook, M.D. (Professional Books, 1988).

Understanding Allergy, Sensitivity and Immunology: A Comprehensive Guide, by Janice V. Joneja, Ph.D., and Leonard Bielory, M.D. (Rutgers University Press, 1994).

Alternative and Natural Health and Healing

The Alternative Health and Medicine Encyclopedia, by James E. Marti (Visible Ink Press, 1995).

Alternative Medicine: The Definitive Guide, by The Burton Goldberg Group (Future Medicine Publishing, Inc., 1994).

The American Holistic Health Association Complete Guide to Alternative Medicine, by William Collinge, M.P.H., Ph.D. (Warner Books, 1996).

Earl Mindell's Herb Bible, by Earl Mindell, M.D. (Simon & Schuster, 1992).

Encyclopedia of Natural Medicine, by Michael Murray, N.D., and J. Pizzarno, N.D. (Prima Publishing, 1991).

Lifetime Treasury of Home Remedies, by Myra Cameron (Parker Publishing Co., Inc., 1993).

Candida-Related Complex

Allergy and Candida Cooking—Rotational Style, by Sondra K. Lewis and Lonnett Blakley (Canary Connect Publications, 1995).

Back to Health: Yeast Control, by Dennis W. Remington, M.D., and Barbara Higa, R.D. (Vitality House International, 1989).

Candida Albicans, by Leon Chaitow, D.O., N.D. (Healing Arts Press, 1988).

The Candida Albicans Yeast-Free Cookbook, by Pat Connolly (Keats Publishing, Inc., 1985).

The Candida Control Cookbook, by Gail Burton (Aslan Publishing, 1993).

The Candida Directory and Cookbook, by Helen Gustafson and Maureen O'Shea (Celestial Arts, 1994).

Candida: A Twentieth Century Disease, by Shirley S. Lorenzani, Ph.D. (Keats Publishing, Inc., 1986).

The Missing Diagnosis, by C. Orian Truss, M.D. (The Missing Diagnosis, 1982).

We Are Not Alone: Learning to Live with Chronic Illness, by Sefra Kobrin Pitzele (Workman Publishing, 1986).

The Yeast Connection Cookbook, by William G. Crook, M.D., and Marjorie Hurt Jones, R.N. (Professional Books, 1989).

The Yeast Connection and the Woman, by William G. Crook (Professional Books, 1995).

The Yeast Syndrome, by John Parks Trowbridge, M.D., and Morton Walker, D.P.M. (Bantam Books, 1986).

Children's Health

Childhood Ear Infections: What Every Parent and Physician Should Know about Prevention, Home Care and Alternative Treatments, by Michael A. Schmidt, M.D. (North Atlantic Books, 1995).

Encyclopedia of Natural Health and Healing for Children, by Marcea Weber, (Prima Publishing, 1994).

Food for Healthy Kids, by Lendon Smith, M.D. (Berkley Publishing, 1985).

Healing Children Naturally, by Michael A. Weiner, Ph.D. (Quantum Books, 1993).

Is This Your Child? Discovering and Treating Unrecognized Allergies, by Doris Rapp, M.D. (William Morrow and Company, Inc., 1992).

Why Your Child Is Hyperactive, by Ben F. Feingold (Random House, 1985).

Chronic Fatigue Syndrome

The Canary and Chronic Fatigue, by Majid Ali (Life Span Press, 1995).

Chronic Fatigue Syndrome and the Yeast Connection, by William G. Crook, M.D. (Professional Books, 1992).

"How to Apply for Social Security Benefits if You Have CFIDS," by Kenneth Casanova. (Available for $4 from the Mass CFIDS Association, 808 Main Street, Waltham, MA 02154.)

Recovering from Chronic Fatigue Syndrome: A Guide to Self-Empowerment, by William Collinge, M.P.H, Ph.D. (Berkley Publications, 1993).

Solving the Puzzle of Chronic Fatigue Syndrome, by Michael Rosenbaum, M.D,. and Murray Susser, M.D. (Life Sciences Press, 1992).

Diet and Nutrition

The Body Ecology Diet: Recovering Your Health and Rebuilding Your Immunity, by Donna Gates and Lynn Schatz (BED Publications, 1993).

Healing Through Nutrition, Melvyn Werbach, M.D. (HarperCollins, 1993).

Jane Brody's Good Food Book, by Jane Brody (Bantam Books, 1987).

Jane Brody's Nutrition Book, by Jane Brody (Bantam Books, 1982).

Nutrition Desk Reference, by Robert H. Garrison and Elizabeth Somer (Keats Publishing, Inc., 1985).

Prescription for Nutritional Healing, by James F. Balch, M.D., and Phyllis A. Balch, C.N.C. (Avery Publishing Group, 1990).

Shopper's Guide to Natural Foods, by the editors of the *East West Journal* (Avery Publishing Group, 1988).

Staying Healthy with Nutrition, by E.M. Haas (Celestial Arts, 1992).

Environmental Health and Illnesses

Chemical Sensitivity: A Guide to Coping with Hypersensitivity Syndrome, Sick Building Syndrome and Other Environmental Illnesses, by Bonnye L. Matthews (McFarland & Co., 1992).

Dentistry without Mercury, by Sam Ziff and Michael F. Ziff (Bio-Probe, 1988).

It's All in Your Head: The Link Between Mercury Amalgams and Illness, by Hal A. Huggins, D.D.S. (Avery Publishing, 1993).

Nontoxic, Natural and Earthwise: How to Protect Yourself and Your Family from Harmful Products and Live in Harmony with the Earth, by Debra Lynn Dadd, G.P. (Putnam's Sons, 1990).

Rapid Guide to Hazardous Chemicals in the Workplace 3rd edition, by Richard J. Lewis, Sr. (Van Nostrand Reinhold, 1994).

Silver Dental Fillings: The Toxic Timebomb, by Sam Ziff (Aurora Press, 1984).

Staying Well in a Toxic World, by Lynn Lawson (The Noble Press, 1993).

The Toxic Labyrinth: A Family's Successful Battle Against Environmental Illness, by Myrna Millar, B. Ed., M.B.A., and Heather Millar, B.S.N., R.N. (Nico Professional Services, Ltd., 1995).

Your Home, Your Health and Well-Being, by David Rousseau, William J. Rea, M.D., and Jean Enwright (Ten Speed Press, 1988).

General Health

Beyond Antibiotics: Fifty (or so) Ways to Boost Immunity and Avoid Antibiotics, by Michael A. Schmidt, M.D., Lendon H. Smith, M.D., and Keith W. Sehnert, M.D. (North Atlantic Books, 1994).

The Doctors Book of Home Remedies, volume I and *The Doctors Book of Home Remedies, volume II*, by Sid Kirschheimer and the editors of *Prevention Magazine* (Bantam Books, 1993 and 1995).

Getting the Most out of Your Vitamins and Minerals, by Jack Challem (Keats Publishing, Inc., 1993).

Good Health Handbook: Hundreds of Tips to Improve Your Health, by the editors of *Consumer Guide* (Publications International, Ltd., 1995).

Great Health Hints and Handy Tips (Reader's Digest General Books, 1994).

Family Health and Medical Guide, by the editors of *Consumer Guide* (Publications International, Ltd., 1994).

The New Wellness Encyclopedia, by the editors of the *University of California at Berkeley Wellness Letter* (Houghton Mifflin Co., 1995).

The PDR Family Guide to Nutrition and Health (Medical Economics, 1995).

The PDR Family Guide to Prescription Drugs (Medical Economics, 1994).

The Vitamin Controversy: Questions and Answers, by E. Cheraskin (Keats Publishing, Inc., 1990).

The Wellness Book, by Herbert Benson, M.D., and Eileen M. Stuart, R.N., M.S. (Simon & Schuster, 1992).

Women's Health

A Woman's Guide to Yeast Infections, by Naomi Baumslag, M.D, and Dia Michels (Pocket Books, 1992).

The Medical Self-Care Book of Women's Health, by B. Hasselbring, S. Greenwood, and M. Castleman (Doubleday & Co., 1987).

The New A to Z of Women's Health: A Concise Encyclopedia, by Christine Ammer (Hunter House, 1989).

The New Our Bodies, Ourselves, by the Boston Women's Health Collective (Simon & Schuster, 1992).

Overcoming Endometriosis, by Mary Lou Ballweg and the Endometriosis Association (Contemporary Books, 1987).

The PDR Family Guide to Women's Health and Prescription Drugs (Medical Economics, 1994).

Premenstrual Syndrome Self-Help Book, by Susan Lark, M.D. (Celestial Arts, 1989).

Unmasking PMS: The Complete Medical Treatment Plan, by Joseph Martorano, M.D., and Maureen Morgan, C.S.W., R.N., with William Fryer (Evans and Company, 1993).

You Don't Have to Live with Cystitis! How to Avoid It—What to Do About It, by Larrian Gillespie (Avon Books, 1988).

Women's Bodies, Women's Wisdom, by Christiane Northrup, M.D. (Bantam Books, 1994).

Support Groups and Organizations

Self-Help Clearinghouses

Self-help clearinghouses are located throughout the United States and help people find and form support and self-help organizations. The list of clearinghouses changes frequently, so for a more updated list or for help finding a clearinghouse near you, contact the American Self-Help Clearinghouse, St. Clares-Riverside Medical Center, Denville, NJ 07834, (201) 625-7101 or the National Self-Help Clearinghouse, Graduate School & University Center, CUNY, Room 620, 25 W. 43rd St., New York, NY 10036, (212) 642-2944.

The American Self-Help Clearinghouse also publishes *The Self-Help Sourcebook*, which lists specific groups throughout the U.S. and offers several helpful chapters on starting support groups. The following list of self-help clearinghouses has been reprinted with permission from the American Self-Help Clearinghouse.

Arizona

Rainy Day People Clearinghouse
P.O. Box 472
Scottsdale, AZ 85252
(602) 231-0868

Arkansas

c/o Helpline (serving northeast
 Arkansas)
P.O. Box 9028
Jonesboro, AR 72403
(501) 932-5555

California

California Self-Help Center
 (statewide)
5839 Green Valley Circle, Suite 100
Culver City, CA 90230
(310) 825-1799 (Monday to Thursday
 10 A.M. to 4 P.M. only)

Connecticut

Connecticut Self-Help/Mutual
 Support Network (statewide)
389 Whitney Ave.
New Haven, CT 06511
(203) 789-7645

Illinois

Self-Help Center (statewide)
Mental Health Association in Illinois
150 Wacher Dr., Suite 900
Chicago, IL 60606
(708) 291-0085 (group information)
(312) 368-9070 (administrative)

Illinois Self-Help Coalition
c/o Wright College, Room 244
3400 N. Austin
Chicago, IL 60634
(312) 481-8837 (administrative)

Macon County Support Group
   Network
c/o Macon County Health
   Department
1221 E. Condit
Decatur, IL 62521
(217) 429-HELP

Self-Help Center
Family Service of Champaign County
405 South State St.
Champaign, IL 61820
(217) 352-0099

Iowa

Iowa Self-Help Clearinghouse
Iowa Pilot Parents, Inc.
33 N. 12th St.
Fort Dodge, IA 50501
(515) 576-5870
(800) 383-4777 (in Iowa only)

Kansas

Self-Help Network (statewide)
Wichita State University, Campus Box
   34
Wichita, KS 67208
(316) 689-3843
(800) 445-0116 (in Kansas only)

Massachusetts

Massachusetts Clearinghouse of
   Mutual Help Groups

Massachusetts Cooperative Extension
University of Massachusetts
113 Skinner Hall
Amherst, MA 01003
(413) 545-2313

Michigan

Michigan Self-Help Clearinghouse
Michigan Protective and Advocacy
   Service
106 W. Allegan, Suite 210
Lansing, MI 48933
(517) 484-7373
(800) 777-5556 (in Michigan only)

Center for Self-Help (Berrien County
   area)
Riverwood Center
P.O. Box 547
Benton Harbor, MI 49022
(616) 925-0594
(800) 336-0341 (in Michigan only)

Minnesota

First Call for Help
166 E. 4th St., Suite 310
St. Paul, MI 55101
(612) 224-1133
(612) 291-8427 (administrative)
*Provides information on existing self-help
   groups statewide.*

Missouri

Support Group Clearinghouse (Kansas
   City area only)
Kansas City Association for Mental
   Health
1009 Baltimore, 5th Floor
Kansas City, MO 64105
(816) 472-HELP
(816) 472-5000 (administrative)

Self-Help Clearinghouse
Greater St. Louis Mental Health
   Association
1905 South Grand
St. Louis, MO 63104
(314) 773-1399

Nebraska

Self-Help Information Services
1601 Euclid Ave.
Lincoln, NE 68502
(402) 476-9668

New Jersey

New Jersey Self-Help Clearinghouse
St. Clares-Riverside Medical Center
Denville, NJ 07834
(201) 625-9565
(800) FOR-MASH (NJ residents only)

New York

Brooklyn Self-Help Clearinghouse
30 Third Ave.
Brooklyn, NY 11217
(718) 875-1420

New York City Self-Help Center
120 West 57th St.
New York, NY 10019
(212) 586-5770

Westchester Self-Help Clearinghouse
456 North St.
White Plains, NY 10605
(914) 949-6301

North Carolina

SupportWorks (greater Mecklenberg
   area)
1018 East Blvd., Suite 5
Charlotte, NC 28203
(704) 331-9500
(704) 377-2055 (administrative)

Ohio

Greater Dayton Self-Help
   Clearinghouse (Dayton area only)
Family Services Association
184 Salem Ave.
Dayton, OH 45406
(513) 225-3004

Greater Toledo Self-Help Network
Harbor Behavioral HealthCare
123 22nd St.
Toledo, OH 43624
(419) 241-6191

Oregon

Northwest Regional Self-Help
   Clearinghouse (includes Seattle,
   WA)
619 Southwest 11th Ave., Room 300
Portland, OR 97205
(503) 222-5555 (information and
   referrals)
(503) 226-9360 (administrative)

Pennsylvania
Self-Help Group Network of the
   Pittsburgh Area
1323 Forbes Ave., Suite 200
Pittsburgh, PA 15219
(412) 261-5363

Self-Help Information Network
   Exchange (S.H.I.N.E.)
c/o Voluntary Action Center
225 N. Washington Ave.
Park Plaza, Lower Level
Scranton, PA 18503
(717) 961-1234

South Carolina

Midland Area Support Group Network
Lexington Medical Center
2720 Sunset Blvd.
West Columbia, SC 29169
(803) 791-9227 (information and
   referrals)
(803) 791-2049 (administrative)

Tennessee

Support Group Clearinghouse
Mental Health Association of Knox
   County
6712 Kingston Pike, #203
Knoxville, TN 37919
(615) 584-6736

Self-Help Clearinghouse
Mental Health Association of
    Memphis
2400 Poplar, Suite 410
Memphis, TN 38112
(901) 323-8485 (information and
    referrals)
(901) 323-0633 (administrative)

Texas

Dallas Self-Help Clearinghouse
Mental Health Association of Dallas
    County
2929 Carlisle, Suite 350
Dallas, TX 75204
(214) 871-2420

Greater San Antonio Self-Help
    Clearinghouse
Mental Health in Greater San Antonio
901 N.E. Loop 410, Suite 500
San Antonio, TX 78209
(512) 826-2288

Self-Help Clearinghouse
Mental Health Association in
    Houston & Harris County
2211 Norfolk, Suite 810
Houston, TX 77098
(713) 523-8963

Tarrant County Self-Help
    Clearinghouse
Mental Health Association of Tarrant
    County
3136 W. 4th St.
Fort Worth, TX 76107
(817) 335-5405

Texas Self-Help Clearinghouse
Mental Health Association in Texas
8401 Shoal Creek Blvd.
Austin, TX 78758
(512) 454-3706

Washington

See Oregon

Washington, DC

Self-Help Clearinghouse of Greater
    Washington (also Northern
    Virginia and Southern Maryland)
Mental Health Association of
    Northern Virginia
7630 Little River Turnpike, Suite 206
Annandale, VA 22003
(703) 941-LINK

Organizations that Offer Information and/or Support

American Council for Headache
    Education
875 Kings Highway, Suite 200
West Deptford, NJ 08096
(800) 255-ACHE

American Dietetic Association
216 W. Jackson Blvd., Suite 800
Chicago, IL 60606
(800) 877-1600
*Provides educational material and
    services that concern nutrition.*

American Foundation for Pain
    Research
120 S. Spalding Dr., Suite 210
Beverly Hills, CA 90212
*Provides information on cystitis,
    endometriosis, and other conditions
    that relate to pelvic pain.*

Candida & Dysbiosis Information
Foundation
P.O. Drawer JF
College Station, TX 77841
(409) 694-8687

Center for Mind/Body Medicine
1110 Camino del Mar, Suite G
Del Mar, CA 92014
(619) 794-2425
(202) 966-7338

Center for Science in the Public
   Interest
Nutrition Action Health Letter
1875 Connecticut Ave. NW, Suite 300
Washington, DC 20009
(202) 332-9110

CFIDS Association
P.O. Box 220398
Charlotte, NC 28222
(714) 362-2343
(800) 442-3437

CFIDS Foundation
965 Mission St., Suite 425
San Francisco, CA 94103
(415) 882-9986

Chemical Sensitivity Disorders
   Association
P.O. Box 24061
Arbutus, MD 21227
(410) 792-4875

Dental Amalgam Mercury Syndrome
   (DAMS)
6025 Osuna Blvd., NE #B
Albuquerque, NM 87109
(505) 888-0111

Ecological Health Organization
P.O. Box 281116
E. Hartford, CT 06128-1116
(203) 528-6235

Endometriosis Association
8585 North 76th Pl.
Milwaukee, WI 53223
(800) 992-3636 in the U.S.
(800) 426-2363 in Canada

Environmental Health Association
1800 S. Robertson Blvd., #380
Los Angeles, CA 90035
(310) 837-2048

Environmental Health Advocacy
   League (ENHALE)
P.O. Box 425
Concord, MA 01742
(508) 287-4543

Environmental Health Network
   (California)
P.O. Box 1155
Larkspur, CA 94977
(415) 331-9804

Environmental Health Network
   (Virginia)
P.O. Box 16267 Gt. Bridge Station
Chesapeake, VA 23328
(804) 424-1162

Environmental Dental Association
9974 Scripps Ranch Blvd., Suite 36
San Diego, CA 92131
(800) 388-8124

Health Research Group
2000 P St., N.W.
Washington, DC 20036
(202) 833-3000

Human Ecology Action League
   (HEAL)
P.O. Box 49126
Atlanta, GA 30359
(404) 248-1898

International Health Foundation
P.O. Box 3494
Jackson, TN 38303
(901) 427-8100

Mass CFIDS Association
808 Main St.
Waltham, MA 02154
(617) 893-4415

National Center for Environmental
   Health Strategies
1100 Rural Ave.
Voorhees, NJ 08043
(609) 429-5358

National CFS Association
919 Scott Ave.
Kansas City, KS 66105
(913) 321-2278

The National Foundation for the
   Chemically Hypersensitive
P.O. Box 9
Wrightsville Beach, NC 28480

The National Headache Foundation
5252 North Western Ave.
Chicago, IL 60625
(800) 843-2256

National Women's Health Network
1325 G St., N.W.
Washington, DC 20005
(202) 347-1140

People's Medical Society
462 Walnut St.
Allentown, PA 18102

The Practical Allergy Research
   Foundation
(800) 787-8780

PMS Access
P.O. Box 9326
Madison, WI
(800) 222-4PMS

Price-Pottenger Nutrition Foundation
   (PPNF)
P.O. Box 2614
La Mesa, CA 91943
(619) 574-7763

Twin Cities Candida Support Group
173 N. McKnight Rd., #204
St. Paul, MN 55119
(612) 578-6606

Well Mind Association
4649 Sunnyside Ave. N.
Seattle, WA 98103
(206) 547-5167

World Research Foundation
153000 Ventura Blvd., Suite 405
Sherman Oaks, CA 91403
(818) 907-5483

Health Hotlines

The Environmental Protection Agency (EPA) has sponsored a pesticide hotline, which provides information on the health hazards of pesticides and helpful information, including how to obtain lab analyses and how to check for toxicity levels around you. The phone number is (800) 858-7378. The EPA also has a lead hotline: (800) LEAD-FYI.

Food and Product Sources

If you plan to order a lot of foods or products by mail, you may want to send a self-addressed stamped envelope for a comprehensive list of available companies and products from the Americans for Safe Foods, 1501 16th Street, NW, Washington, DC 20036. Another great source is the *Allergy Products Directory* (APD), which contains more than one thousand sources for specialty foods. For a directory, send a self-addressed stamped envelope to Allergy Products Directory, P.O. Box 640, Menlo Park, CA 94026.

Product Sources

Allergy Alternative
526 Shagbark St.
Windsor, CA 95492
(800) 838-1514
Offers a diverse line of environmentally safe products at discounted prices, including personal-care products, cosmetics, household cleaning products, vitamins, antifungal products, and acidophilus.

Allergy Research Group/NutriCology
Inc.
400 Preda St.
San Leandro, CA 94577
(800) 545-9960
Offers vitamins, minerals, amino acid products, glandulars, probiotics, and specialty products.

Cardiovascular Research/Ecological
Formulas
1061 B Shary Circle
Concord, CA 94518
(800) 888-4585
Offers vitamins and nutritional products.

College Pharmacy
833 N. Tejon St.

Colorado Springs, CO 80903
(800) 888-9358
Can fill prescriptions for antifungal medicines.

Freeda Vitamins
36 East 41st St.
New York, NY 10017
(800) 777-3737
Manufactures and sells yeast-free vitamins, minerals, and other supplies.

Klaire Laboratories/Vital Life
1573 W. Seminole
San Marcos, CA 92069
(800) 533-7255
Offers over one hundred products, including vitamins, amino acids products, and Vita Plex and Vita Dophilus (two hypoallergenic brands of acidophilus).

L&H Vitamins
3233 47th Ave.
Long Island City, NY 11101
(800) 221-1152
Sells a wide variety of vitamins and herbal and nutritional supplements at discount prices.

275

National CFIDS Buyer's Club
1187 Coast Village Rd., #1-280
Santa Barbara, CA 93108
(800) 366-6056
Publishes a quarterly newsletter and offers a wide variety of vitamins and nutritional supplements at discount prices.

Nature's Sunshine Products, Inc.
75 E. 1700 S.
P.O. Box 19005
Provo, UT 84605
(801) 342-4300
Offers herbs and nutritional supplements.

Natural Lifestyle Supplies
16 Lookout Dr.
Asheville, NC 28804
(704) 254-9606
Offers natural foods, products, and books for people with environmental illnesses.

Nature's Way Products, Inc.
10 Mountain Springs Parkway
Springville, UT 84663
(800) 453-1468
Offers nutritional products, including herbs and its own line of vitamins.

National Ecological and
  Environmental Delivery System
  (NEEDS)
527 Charles Ave., Suite 12-A
Syracuse, NY 13209
(800) 634-1380
Offers a wide variety of products for chemically sensitive people, including household products, cosmetics, appliances, supplements, and other supplies.

Wellness Health Pharmaceuticals
2800 S. 18th St.
Birmingham, AL 35209
(800) 227-2627
Can fill bulk prescriptions.

Food Sources

Arrowhead Mills
P.O. Box 2059
Hereford, TX 79045
(800) 749-0730 (to order a mail-order catalog)
Carries a variety of natural and organic products and whole foods, cereals, vegetable oils, as well as wheat- and gluten-free flours.

Community Alliance with Family
  Farmers
P.O. Box 464
Davis, CA 95617
(916) 756-8518
Offers the National Organic Directory, *a complete list of organic wholesalers around the U.S. and companies that sell organic foods.*

Eden Acres
Organic Network
12100 Lima Center Rd.
Clinton, MI 49236
(517) 456-4288

Has a 150-page directory of suppliers of organic meats, fruits, and vegetables.

Harvest Direct, Inc.
P.O. Box 988
Knoxville, TN 37901
(800) 835-2867
Sells over five hundred foods and products that focus on a vegetarian lifestyle.

The Organic Foods Trade Association
P.O. Box 1078
Greenfield, MA 01302
(413) 774-7511
Supplies information about companies that sell organic foods.

Special Foods
9207 Shotgun Ct.
Springfield, VA 22153
(703) 644-0991
Offers products formulated for people with food allergies, chemical sensitivities, and mold allergies. Products include breads, flours, nut butters, baking powders, crackers, cookies, and pastas.

Physicians Who Treat CRC

Below are definitions of some of the most commonly used professional credentials:

D.C.	Doctor of Chiropractic	**N.D.**	Doctor of Naturopathy
D.O.	Doctor of Osteopathy	**O.M.D.**	Oriental Medical Doctor
H.M.D.	Homeopathic Medical Doctor	**Ph.D.**	Doctor of Philosophy
M.D.	Doctor of Medicine	**R.N.**	Registered Nurse

This list is arranged alphabetically by state and then by area code. The authors would like to thank the American Academy of Environmental Medicine (AAEM) and the Price-Pottenger Nutrition Foundation (PPNF) for their help. If this list does not help you locate a physician in your area, there are several other sources through which you may be able to find medical help:

- For a list of physicians who treat CRC in your area, send a self-addressed stamped envelope to the International Health Foundation, P.O. Box 3494, Jackson, TN, 38303. Their phone number is (901) 427-8100.

- For a list of nutrition-oriented health-care providers in your area, send a self-addressed stamped envelope and $6 to the Price-Pottenger Nutrition Foundation, P.O. Box 2614, La Mesa, CA 91943-2614. Be sure to specify the desired state and a neighboring state if your city is near the border.

- For names of physicians who practice environmental medicine in your area, send $3 and a self-addressed stamped envelope to the American Academy of Environmental Medicine, P.O. Box 16106, Denver, CO 80216.

- For names of naturopathic physicians, call or write the American Association of Naturopathic Physicians, 2366 E. Lake Avenue E, Suite 322, Seattle, WA 98102, (206) 323-7610.

- For names of homeopathic physicians in your area call or write the National Center for Homeopathy, 801 N. Fairfax St., Suite 306, Alexandria, VA 22314, (703) 548-7790 or the International Foundation for Homeopathy, 2366 E. Lake Avenue E, Suite 301, Seattle, WA 98102, (206) 324-8230.

- Pick up a copy of the *Alternative Medicine Yellow Pages* published by Future Medical Publishing and available at your local library or bookstore.

- Two laboratories that do blood and stool tests for Candida and that may be able to refer you to a physician in your area are Meridan Labs at (206) 631-8922 and Great Smokies Lab Client Services at (800) 522-4762.

- Two other ways to find physicians who treat CRC are through inquiries at your local health food store or by contacting environmental illness-related self-help groups in your area.

Alabama

Area Code 205
Andrew M. Brown, M.D.
515 S. Third St.
Gadsen, AL 35901
(205) 547-4971
(800) 872-7304

Gus J. Prosch, M.D.
759 Valley St.
Birmingham, AL 35226
(205) 823-6180

Alaska

Area Code 907
Sandra C. Denton, M.D.
3201 C St., Suite 306
Anchorage, AK 99503
(907) 563-6200

Robert J. Rowen, M.D.
615 E. 82nd St., Suite 300
Anchorage, AK 99518
(907) 344-7775

Arizona

Area Code 602
Ralph F. Herro, M.D.
5115 N. Central Ave.
Phoenix, AZ 85012
(602) 266-2374

Stanley R. Olsztyn, M.D. (H)
4350 E. Camelback Rd., Suite B-220
Phoenix, AZ 85018
(602) 840-8424

Arkansas

Area Code 501
Harold H. Hedges, M.D.
424 N. University
Little Rock, AR 72205
(501) 664-4810

Aubrey M. Worrell, M.D.
3900 Hickory St.
Pine Bluff, AR 71603
(501) 535-8200

California

Area Code 209
Stockmann Chiropractic Center
Ralph Stockmann, D.C.
555 W. Benjamin Holt Drive, #410
Stockton, CA 95207
(209) 951-7864

Area Code 213
Albert A. Hertz, D.C.
415 3/4 N. Larchmont Blvd.
Los Angeles, CA 90004
(213) 461-9373

Area Code 310
James P. Blumenthal, D.C.
1619 1/2 Montana Ave.
Santa Monica, CA
(310) 451-3683

Theresa Dale, Ph.D., N.D.
23410 Civic Center Way, Suite E-11
Malibu, CA 90265
(310) 317-4441

Keith DeOrio, M.D.
1821 Wilshire Blvd., Suite 100
Santa Monica, CA
(310) 828-3096

Jesse Lynn Hanley, M.D.
22917 Pacific Coast Highway,
    Suite 220
Malibu, CA 90265
(310) 465-9393

Huy Hoang, M.D.
12732 Washington Blvd., Suite D
Los Angeles, CA 90066
(310) 822-4614
    and
1010 Crenshaw Blvd., Suite 170
Torrance, CA 90501
(310) 320-1132

Cathie-Ann Lippman, M.D.
291 S. La Cienega Blvd., Suite 207
Beverly Hills, CA 90211
(310) 289-8430

David J. Nickel, O.M.D.
1530 Lincoln Blvd., Suite D
Santa Monica, CA 90401
(310) 396-0175

Marvin Portner, M.D.
910 Via De La Paz, #205
Pacific Palisades, CA 90272
(310) 454-6226

Murray R. Susser, M.D.
2730 Wilshire Blvd., #110
Santa Monica, CA 90403
(310) 453-4424

Area Code 408
Randy S. Baker, M.D.
2955 Park Ave.
Soquel, CA 95073
(408) 476-1886

Daniel Beilin, O.M.D.
9057 Soquel Dr., A-B
Aptos, CA 95003
(408) 685-1125

Area Code 415
Elson M. Haas, M.D.
25 Mitchell Blvd., Suite 8
San Rafael, CA 94903
(415) 472-2343

Vincent A. Mark, M.D.
4145 Clares St., #F
Capitola, CA 95010
(408) 462-2838

John C. Wakefield, M.D.
18988 Cox Ave., Suite D
Saratoga, CA 95070
(408) 366-0660

Area Code 415
Robert F. Cathcart, M.D.
127 Second St.
Los Altos, CA 94022
(415) 949-2822

Ellen Cutler, D.C.
770 Tamalpuis Dr., Suite 203
Corte Madera, CA 94925
(415) 924-2273

Vadim I. Kvitash, M.D., Ph.D.
2299 Post St., #306
San Francisco, CA 94117
(415) 771-5726

Paul Lynn, M.D.
345 W. Portal Ave.
San Francisco, CA 94127
(415) 566-1000

Vincent A. Marinkovich, M.D.
90 Middlefield Rd., #100
Menlo Park, CA 94027
(415) 327-8380

Claude J. Marquette, M.D.
5050 El Camino Real, #110
Los Altos, CA 94022
(415) 964-6700

Area Code 510
Cecil A. Bradley, M.D.
2191 Mowry Ave., Suite 500H
Fremont, CA 94538
(510) 783-9900

Alan S. Charles, M.D.
1414 Maria Ln.
Walnut Creek, CA 94596
(510) 937-3331

Don Canavan, N.D.
555 Pierce St., #724
Albany, CA 94706
(510) 524-8652

Geraldine P. Donaldson, M.D.
1074 Murrieta Blvd.
Livermore, CA 94550
(510) 443-8282

Steven H. Gee, M.D.
595 Estudillo Ave.
San Leandro, CA 94577
(510) 483-5881

Stephen Langer, M.D.
3031 Telegraph Ave.
Berkeley, CA 94705
(510) 548-7384

Betty Stratford, M.D.
Mary Lou Toraason, M.D.
1501 Bollinger Canyon Rd.
San Ramon, CA 94583
(510) 837-3911

John P. Toth, M.D.
2299 Bacon St., Suite 10
Concord, CA 94520
(510) 682-5660

Area Code 619
Allergy Medical Group of San Diego,
    Inc.
Milan L. Brandon, M.D.
2800 Third Ave.
San Diego, CA 92103
(619) 291-2321

Lance L. Clothey, D.C.
7125 El Cajon Blvd., #3
San Diego, CA 92115
(619) 465-4880

Francois Joseph Durand, M.D.,
    H.M.D.
353 3rd Ave., #202
Chula Vista, CA 91910
(800) 867-2307

Mai Solange Durand, M.D., H.M.D.
353 3rd Ave., #202
Chula Vista, CA 91910
(800) 867-2307

Kathi Head, N.D.
2496 E St., Suite 300
San Diego, CA 92102
(619) 236-8285

John A. Henderson, M.D.
2055 Third Ave.
San Diego, CA 92101
(619) 239-7747

Ronald M. Lesko, D.O., M.P.H.
13983 Mango Dr., #103
Del Mar, CA 92014
(619) 259-2444

Antonio E. J. Monti, M.D., F.A.A.F.P.
505 North Mollison Ave., #202
El Cajon, CA 92021
(619) 588-4949

Charles A. Moss, M.D.
8950 Villa La Jolla Dr., Suite 2162
La Jolla, CA 92037
(619) 457-1314

Ron R. Romero, D.C.
2147 Newcastle Ave.
Cardiff, CA 92007
(619) 942-2733

Andrew W. Specht, D.C.
230 Second St., #101
Encinitas, CA 92024
(619) 632-0098

Jack Stone, D.C.
8870 La Mesa Blvd.
La Mesa, CA 91941
(619) 463-1199

Joseph Watson, D.O.
1330 Camino Del Mar
Del Mar, CA 92014
(619) 792-2635

William Welles, D.C.
6565 Balboa Ave., #A
San Diego, CA 92111
(619) 541-1440

Erhardt Zinke, M.D.
2131 Winter Warm Rd.
Fallbrook, CA 92028
(619) 728-4901

Area Code 707
Hill Park Clinic
Brian Bouch, M.D.
245 Kentucky St., #A
Petaluma, CA 94952
(707) 778-3171

Peter V. Madill, M.D.
7005 Hazel Cotter Ct., #3
Sebastopol, CA 95472
(707) 823-3312

Area Code 714
Marc D. Braunstein, D.O.
24541 Pacific Park Dr., Suite 103
Aliso Viejo, CA 92656
(714) 362-2121

Raymond J. Bunch, D.C.
8780 Warner Ave., Suite 8
Fountain Valley, CA 92708
(714) 375-0552

Health Dynamics
Howard Cohn, D.C., Bob Heron, D.C.
Guy Huston, D.C., Albert Lee, D.C.
Greg Olsen, D.C.
3200 Bristol St., Suite 695
Costa Mesa, CA 92626
(714) 668-1112

Area Code 805
H. J. Hoegerman, M.D.
101 W. Arrellaga
Santa Barbara, CA 93101
(805) 963-1824

Dominique Manasson, D.C.
300 S. Fifth St., Suite C
Oxnard, CA 93030
(805) 483-6636

Dale Migliaccio, D.C.
1725 State St.
Santa Barbara, CA 93101
(805) 687-4515

Robert G. Morris, M.S., D.C.
708 Cuyama Rd.
Ojai, CA 93023
(805) 640-8814

Timothy Tupper, D.C.
4173 State St.
Santa Barbara, CA 93110
(805) 683-8884

Area Code 818
Allergy & Nutrition Clinic
James Privitera, M.D.
105 N. Grandview Ave.
Covina, CA 91723
(818) 966-1618

Douglas Hunt, M.D.
2625 Alameda
Burbank, CA 91505
(818) 566-9889

N. Rowan Richards, D.C., D.A.B.C.I.
1230 Huntington Dr., Suite 10
Duarte, CA 91010
(818) 303-5567

Area Code 909
Tri-City Chiropractic Clinic
Donn D. Fisher, D.C.
100 Pierre Rd.
Walnut, CA 91789
(909) 594-6181

Judi G. Milin, D.C.
55450 S. Circle Dr.
P.O. Box 3157
Idyllwild, CA 92549
(909) 659-4522

Kenneth Pramann, D.C.
P.O. Box 297
Big Bear City, CA 92314
(909) 585-2400

Area Code 916
Stephen Banister, M.D.
11325 Varnell Dr.
Nevada City, CA 95959
(916) 265-4574

Dennis K. Crawford, D.C.
10231 Fair Oaks Blvd.
Fair Oaks, CA 95628
(916) 962-3101

Michael J. Kwiker, D.O.
3301 Alta Arden, #3
Sacramento, CA 95825
(916) 489-4400

Sunil P. Perera, M.D.
404 Sunrise Ave.
Roseville, CA 95661
(916) 782-7758
   and
1 Scripps Dr., Suite 105
Sacramento, CA 95825
(916) 925-1056

James F. Ransdell, M.D.
635 Anderson Rd., #2
Davis, CA 95616
(916) 756-0131

Bessie Jo Tillman, M.D.
2054 Market St.
Redding, CA 96001
(916) 246-3022
(916) 246-7894

Colorado

Area Code 303
Kendall A. Gerdes, M.D.
Two Steele St., #200
Denver, CO 80206
(303) 377-8837

Area Code 719
Springs Health Clinic
James R. Fish, M.D.
3030 N. Hancock Ave.
Colorado Springs, CO 80907
(719) 471-2273

Area Code 970
Rob Krakovitz, M.D.
430 W. Main St.
Aspen, CO 81611
(970) 927-4394

Connecticut

Area Code 203
Sidney M. Baker, M.D.
40 Hillside Rd. N.
Weston, CT 06883
(203) 227-8444

Alan M. Dattner, M.D.
370 Riverside Dr.
North Grosvenordale, CT 06255
(203) 923-9596

Center for Health
Enrico Liva, N.D.
Jacqueline Germain, N.D.
Keli Samuelson, N.D.
Michael Kane, N.D.
87 Bernie O'Rourke Dr.
Middletown, CT 06457
(203) 347-8600

Robban A. Sica, M.D.
325 Boston Post Rd.
Orange, CT 06477
(203) 799-7733

Area Code 860
Jerrold N. Finnie, M.D.
333 Kennedy Dr., #L-204
Torrington, CT 06790
(860) 489-8977

Delaware

Area Code 302
Jerry Groll, M.D.
421 Savannah Rd.
Lewes, DE 19958
(302) 645-2833

Florida

Area Code 305
Ervin Barr, D.O.
2350 W. Oakland Park Blvd., #90
Fort Lauderdale, FL 33311
(305) 731-8080

Martin Brody, M.D.
7150 W. 20th Ave., #312
Hialeah, FL 33016
(305) 822-9035

Stanley J. Cannon, M.D.
9085 S.W. 87th Ave.
Miami, FL 33176
(305) 279-3020

Institute of Natural Medicine
Fariss Kimbell, M.D.
3400 Park Central Blvd. N, #3450
Pompano Beach, FL 33064
(305) 977-3700

Barry M. Seinfeld, M.D.
16800 N.W. 2nd Ave.
Parkway Medical Plaza, Suite 301
North Miami Beach, FL 33169
(305) 652-1062

Area Code 407
Roy Kupsinel, M.D.
P.O. Box 620550
Oviedo, FL 32762
(407) 365-6681

Albert F. Robbins, D.O.
400 S. Dixie Highway
Bldg. 2, Suite 210
Boca Raton, FL 33432
(407) 395-3282

Area Code 813
Ray C. Wunderlich, Jr., M.D.
666 Sixth St. S, Suite 206
St. Petersburg, FL 33701
(813) 822-3612

Area Code 904
Hana T. Chaim, D.O.
595 W. Granada Blvd., Suite D
Ormond Beach, FL 32174
(904) 672-9000

Georgia

Area Code 404
Stephen B. Edelson, M.D., F.A.A.F.P.,
F.A.A.E.M.
3833 Roswell Rd., Suite 110
Atlanta, GA 30342
(404) 841-0088

Milton Fried, M.D.
4426 Tilly Mill Rd.
Atlanta, GA 30360
(404) 451-4857

Bernard Mlaver, M.D.
4480 N. Shallowford Rd., Suite 222
Atlanta, GA 30338
(404) 395-1600

Area Code 706
Otis J. Woodard, M.D.
Healthspan Clinic
P.O. Box 806
Clayton, GA 30525
(706) 782-1219

Hawaii

Area Code 808
George M. Ewing, M.D.
1329 Lusitana St., #603
Honolulu, HI 96813
(808) 521-2712

Douglas A. Miller, M.D.
400 Hualani St., Suite 191-B
Hilo, HI 96720
(808) 961-5700

Idaho

Area Code 208
Holistic Naturopathic Center
5920 N. Government Way, #6
Coeur D'Alene, ID 83814
(208) 772-9502

Illinois

Area Code 217
W. Robert Elghammer, M.D.
723 N. Logan Ave.
Danville, IL 61832
(217) 446-3259

Guy O. Pfeiffer, M.D.
R.R. 3, Box 283
Mattoon, IL 61938
(217) 235-3822

Area Code 309
Midwest Health Renewal Center
Thomas Hesselink, M.D.
205 S. Englewood Dr.
Metamora, IL 61548
(309) 367-2321

Area Code 618
Corzine Chiropractic Office
James Corzine, D.C.
210 W. Market St.
Christopher, IL 62822
(618) 724-9200

Area Code 630
Thomas Hesselink, M.D.
888 S. Edgelawn Dr.
Aurora, IL 60506
(630) 844-0011

Area Code 708
Robert W. Boxer, M.D.
64 Old Orchard Rd.
Skokie, IL 60077
(708) 677-0260

Paul J. Dunn, M.D.
715 Lake St., #106
Oak Park, IL 60301
(708) 383-3800

Richard E. Hrdlicka, M.D.
302 Randal Rd., #206
Geneva, IL 60134
(708) 232-1900

Joseph M. Mercola, D.O.
1443 W. Schaumburg
Schaumburg, IL 60194
(708) 980-1777

George E. Shambaugh, Jr., M.D.
40 S. Clay St.
Hinsdale, IL 60521
(708) 887-1130

Thomas L. Stone, M.D.
1811 Hicks Rd.
Rolling Meadows, IL 60008
(708) 934-1100

Area Code 815
Gary R. Oberg, M.D.
31 N. Virginia St.
Crystal Lake, IL 60014
(815) 455-1990

Indiana

Area Code 219
Thomas G. Goodwin, M.D.
6111 Harrison St., #343 M.C.
Merrillville, IN 46410
(219) 980-6117

Michael Holton, M.D.
3217 Lake Ave.
Fort Wayne, IN 46805
(219) 422-9471

Area Code 317
Robert M. Armer, M.D.
8803 N. Meridian St., #340
Indianapolis, IN 46260
(317) 846-7341

Terry F. Garcia, M.D.
3266 N. Meridian St.
Indianapolis, IN 46260
(317) 931-0243

Iowa

Area Code 319
Nyle D. Kauffman, M.D.
2460 Towncrest Dr.
Iowa City, IA 52240
(319) 338-7862

Kansas

Area Code 316
Center for Healing Arts
Hugh D. Riordan, M.D.
3100 N. Hillside Ave.
Wichita, KS 67219
(316) 682-3100

Charles T. Hinshaw, Jr., M.D.
1833 N. Rock Rd.
Wichita, KS 67206
(316) 685-4622

Kentucky

Area Code 502
Morgan Medical Clinic
Kirk D. Morgan, M.D.
9105 U.S. Highway 42
Prospect, KY 40059
(502) 228-0156

Nanine S. Henderson, D.O.
4010 Dupont Circle, #200
St. Matthews, KY 40207
(502) 893-5422

Louisiana

Area Code 504
Stephanie F. Cave, M.D.
7777 Hennessy, Suite 101
Baton Rouge, LA 70808
(504) 767-7433

Maine

Area Code 207
Environmental Health Center of
  Maine
Ray Psonak, D.O.
27 Date St.
Old Orchard Beach, ME 04064
(207) 934-2216

Women to Women
1 Pleasant St.
Yarmouth, ME 04096
(207) 846-6163

Maryland

Area Code 301
James H. Brodsky, M.D.
4701 Willard Ave., #224
Chevy Chase, MD 20815
(301) 652-6760

Barbara A. Solomon, M.D.
8109 Harford Rd.
Baltimore, MD 21234
(301) 668-5611

Area Code 410
Richard E. Layton, M.D.
901 Dulaney Valley Rd., Suite 602
Towson, MD 21204
(410) 337-2707

Massachusetts

Area Code 413
Barry D. Elson, M.D.
52 Maplewood Shops
Old South St.
Northampton, MA 01060
(413) 584-7787

Keenan & O'Neil
Joseph P. Keenan, M.D.
75 Springfield Rd.
Westfield, MA 01085
(413) 568-2304

R. Gopal Malladi, M.D.
1221 Main St.
Cath. Horan Medical Bldg.
Holyoke, MA 01040
(413) 536-2978

Area Code 508
Michael Janson, M.D.
275 Millway, Box 732
Barnstable, MA 02630
(508) 362-4343

N. Thomas La Cava, M.D.
360 West Boylston St., Suite 107
West Boylston, MA 01583
(508) 854-1380

Area Code 617
Kenneth J. Emonds, Ph.D.
New England Center for
   Environmental Medicine
Newbury, MA 01951
(617) 465-5009

Carol Englender, M.D.
1126 Beacon St.
Newton, MA 02161
(617) 965-7770

Michigan

Area Code 313
Edward J. Conley, D.O.
G3494 Beecher Rd.
Flint, MI 48532
(313) 230-8677

Paula G. Davey, M.D., M.T.
425 E. Washington, Suite 201
Ann Arbor, MI 48104
(313) 662-3384

Nedra Downing, D.O.
5639 Sashabaw Rd.
Clarkston, MI 48346
(313) 625-6677

Gerald Keyte, D.O.
29830 Ford Rd.
Garden City, MI 48135
(313) 522-0667

Area Code 616
Born Preventive Health Care Clinic
Grant R. Born, D.O., and Tammy
   Geurkink, D.O.
2687 44th St. S.E.
Grand Rapids, MI 49512
(616) 455-3550

Area Code 810
Gerald Natzke, D.O., A.A.E.M.,
   A.A.O.A.
1044 Gilbert Rd.
Flint, MI 48532
(810) 733-3140

Minnesota

Area Code 612
Michelle I. Ansorge, M.D.
Southwest Clinic
6121 Woodale Ave. S.
Edina, MN 55424
(612) 920-6000

William Christian, M.D.
Southwest Clinic
6121 Woodale Ave. S.
Edina, MN 55424
(612) 920-6000

Jean R. Eckerly, M.D.
10700 Old City Rd. 15, #350
Minneapolis, MN 55441
(612) 593-9458

Keith W. Sehnert, M.D.
6200 Excelsior Blvd., #104
St. Louis Park, MN 55416
(612) 920-0102

Missouri

Area Code 314
Rolf E. Gryte, D.O.
Osage Beach Allergy Clinic
Neis Medical Center
106 Parkway Center
Osage Beach, MO 65065
(314) 348-6733
(314) 348-3001

Madeline Permutt, D.C.
9401 Grandview Dr.
St. Louis, MO 63132
(314) 997-2111

Tipu Sultan, M.D.
Allergy Treatment Center
11585 W. Florissant Rd.
Florissant, MO 63033
(314) 921-5600

Harvey Walker, Jr., M.D., Ph.D.
Preventive Medicine, Inc.
138 N. Meramec Ave.
St. Louis, MO 63105
(314) 721-7227

Area Code 816
Applewood Medical Center
Lawrence E. Dorman, D.O.
9120 E. 35th St. S.
Independence, MO 64052
(816) 358-2712

James L. Rowland, D.O.
8133 Wornall Rd.
Kansas City, MO 64114
(816) 361-4077

Montana

Area Code 406
Curt G. Kurtz, M.D.
300 N. Willson Ave., #502E
Bozeman, MT 59715
(406) 587-5561

Catherine H. Steele, M.D.
2509 7th Ave. S.
Great Fallls, MT 59405
(406) 727-4757

Nevada

Area Code 702
Allergy Institute of Nevada
Reed W. Hyde, M.D.
2225 E. Flamingo Rd., #301
Las Vegas, NV 89119
(702) 731-3117

Center of Advanced Medicine
Robert Bliss Vance, D.O., H.M.D.
801 S. Rancho Dr., #F2
Las Vegas, NV 89106
(702) 385-7771

Gerber Medical Clinic
Michael L. Gerber, M.D.
3670 Grant Dr., #101
Reno, NV 89509
(702) 826-1900

Nevada Clinic
Daniel F. Royal, M.D.
3720 Howard Hughes Pkwy.
Las Vegas, NV 89109
(702) 732-1400

New Hampshire

Area Code 603
Michele C. Moore, M.D.
115 Key Rd.
Keene, NH 03431
(603) 357-2180

New Jersey

Area Code 201
Constance Alfano, M.D.
104 Chestnut St.
Ridgewood, NJ 07450
(201) 444-4622

Majid Ali, M.D.
95 E. Main St.
Denville, NJ 07834
(201) 586-4111

Faina Munits, M.D.
51Pleasant Valley Way
West Orange, NJ 07052
(201) 736-3743

Area Code 609
Magaziner Medical Center
Allan Magaziner, D.O., P.C.
1907 Greentree Rd.
Cherry Hill, NJ 08003
(609) 424-8222

Area Code 908
Allergy & Asthma Assn.
Richard Podell, M.D.
571 Central Ave., #106
New Providence, NJ 07974
(908) 464-3800

William T. Kelly, D.C.
525 Highway 70, #A6
Lakewood, NJ 08701
(908) 370-8160

New Mexico

Area Code 505
Jacqueline Krohn, M.D.
Los Alamos Medical Center, #136
Los Alamos, NM 87544
(505) 662-9620

Ralph J. Luciani, D.O.
2301 San Pedro N.E., Suite G
Albuquerque, NM 87110
(505) 888-5995

Shirley B. Scott, M.D.
P.O. Box 2670
Santa Fe, NM 87504
(505) 986-9960

W. A. Shrader, Jr., M.D.
141 Paseo De Peralta, Suite A
Santa Fe Center for Allergy and
   Environmental Medicine
Santa Fe, NM 87501
(505) 983-8890

New York

Area Code 212
Leo Galland, M.D.
133 E. 73rd St.
New York, NY 10021
(212) 861-9000

Robert M. Giller, M.D.
960 Park Ave.
New York, NY 10028
(212) 472-2002

Ronald L. Hoffman, M.D.
40 E. 30th St.
New York, NY 10016
(212) 779-1744

Warren M. Levin, M.D.
Physicians for Complementary
   Medicine
24 W. 57th St., Suite 701
New York, NY 10019
(212) 397-5900

Albert Nehl, N.D.
10th St. Chiropractic
15 E. 10th St.
New York, NY 10003
(212) 982-4449
   and
c/o Life Quest, Inc.
P.O. Box 129
Kingston, GA 30145
(770) 336-5521

Morton M. Teich, M.D.
930 Park Ave.
New York, NY 10028
(212) 988-1821

Area Code 315
Sherry A. Rogers, M.D.
2800 W. Genesee St., Box 2716
Syracuse, NY 13220
(315) 488-2856

The Wellness Institute
Robert W. Snider, M.D.
284 Andrew St.
Massena, NY 13662
(315) 764-7328

Area Code 516
Joseph D. Beasley, M.D.
221 Broadway, Suite 303
Amityville, NY 11701
(516) 598-2960

Christopher L. Calapai, D.O.
1900 Hempstead Tpke.
East Meadow, NY 11554
(516) 794-0404

Mitchell Kurk, M.D.
310 Broadway
Lawrence, NY 11559
(516) 239-5540

Area Code 518
Lynn M. Allison, D.C.
20 Front St.
Ballston Spa, NY 12020
(518) 884-9395

Area Code 716
Kalpana D. Patel, M.D.
65 Wehrie Dr.
Buffalo, NY 14225
(716) 837-1320
(716) 833-2213

Area Code 718
I-Tsu Chao, M.D.
1641 E. 18th St.
Brooklyn, NY 11229
(718) 998-3331

Pavel Yutis, M.D.
1309 W. 7th St.
Brooklyn, NY 11204
(718) 259-2122

Area Code 914
Neil L. Block, M.D., A.A.F.P.
60 Dutchhill Rd.
Orangeburg, NY 10962
(914) 359-3300

Steven Bock, M.D.
Rhinebeck Health Center
108 Montgomery St.
Rhinebeck, NY 12572
(914) 876-7082

Alfred V. Zamm, M.D.
111 Maiden Ln.
Kingston, NY 12401
(914) 338-7766

North Carolina

Area Code 704
F. Keels Dickson, M.D.
485 N. Wendover Rd.
Charlotte, NC 28211
(704) 366-7921
(800) 704-0206

Flechas Family Practice
Jorge Flechas, M.D.
724 5th Ave. W.
Hendersonville, NC 28739
(704) 693-3015

Area Code 910
Walter A. Ward, M.D.
1411-B Plaza West Rd.
Winston-Salem, NC 27114
(910) 760-0240

North Dakota

Area Code 701
Brian E. Briggs, M.D.
718 6th St. S.W.
Minot, ND 58701
(701) 838-6011

Richard H. Leigh, M.D.
2314 Library Circle
Grand Forks, ND 58201
(701) 775-5527

Ohio

Area Code 216
Donald S. Nelson, M.D.
Francis J. Waickman, M.D.
Michael Waickman, M.D.
544 White Pond Dr., Suite B
Akron, OH 44320
(216) 867-3767

Preventive Medicine Group
Derrick Lonsdale, M.D.
24700 Center Ridge Rd., #317
Cleveland, OH 44145
(216) 835-0104

Area Code 419
L. Terry Chappell, M.D.
Jay Nielsen, M.D.
122 Thurman St., Box 207
Bluffton, OH 45817
(419) 358-4627

Charles S. Resseger, D.O.
853 S. Norwalk Rd., P.O. Box 374
Norwalk, OH 44857
(419) 668-9615

Area Code 513
Richard F. Bahr, M.D.
383 Regency Ridge
Centerville, OH 45459
(513) 435-2101

John H. Boyles, Jr., M.D.
7076 Corporate Way
Centerville, OH 45459
(513) 434-0555

Heather Morgan, M.D.
138 S. Main St.
Centerville, OH 45458
(513) 439-1797

Charles W. Platt, M.D.
552 S. West St.
Versailles, OH 45380
(513) 526-3271

Area Code 614
Sandra M. Stewart-Pinkham, M.D.
2170 Riverside Dr.
Columbus, OH 43221
(614) 488-8256

Oklahoma

Area Code 405
Richard B. Dawson, M.D.
4805 S. Western
Oklahoma City, OK 73109
(405) 528-2051
   and
707 N.W. 13th St.
Oklahoma City, OK 73103
(405) 636-1506

Howard E. Hagglund, M.D.
2227 W. Lindsey, #1401
Norman, OK 73069
(405) 329-4457

William H. Philpott, M.D.
17171 S.E. 29th St.
Choctaw, OK 73020
(405) 390-3009
Specializes in magnetic therapy.

Area Code 918
Anderson Clinic
Leon Anderson, D.O.
121 S. 2nd St.
Jenks, OK 74037
(918) 299-5038

Oregon

Area Code 503
John E. Gambee, M.D.
66 Club Rd., #140
Eugene, OR 97401
(503) 686-2536

Debra G. Green, M.D.
John A. Green III, M.D.
117 N.E. Third Ave.
Canby, OR 97013
(503) 266-7933

Health Education Corporation
Richard Brouse, D.C.
8800 S.E. Sunnyside Rd., #111
Clackamus, OR 97015
(503) 654-3225

Richard M. Noble, M.D.
11270 N.W. Reeves St.
Portland, OR 97229
(503) 626-6614

Ronald L. Peters, M.D., M.P.H
1607 Siskiyou Blvd.
Ashland, OR 97520
(503) 482-7007

K. Rifkin, N.D.
338 2nd St.
Lake Oswego, OR 97034
(503) 636-2975

Area Code 541
Cascade Chiropractic Center
Jim Wilkens, D.C., C.C.S.P.
477 N.E. Greenwood Ave.
Bend, OR 97701
(541) 382-8866

Paul E. Dart, M.D.
3495 Harris St.
Eugene, OR 97405
(541) 484-7202

Pennsylvania

Area Code 215
Harold E. Buttram, M.D.
5724 Clymer Rd.
Quakertown, PA 18951
(215) 536-1890

Leland J. Green, M.D.
P.O. Box 508
Lansdale, PA 19446
(215) 855-9501

Conrad G. Maulfair, Jr., D.O.
1413 State St.
Mertztown, PA 19539
(800) 733-4065

New Life Center
P. Jayalakshmi, M.D.
K. R. Sampathachar, M.D.
6366 Sherwood Rd.
Philadelphia, PA 19151
(215) 473-4226
    and
330 Breezewood Rd.
Lehighton, PA 18235
(215) 473-4226

Area Code 412
Ear, Nose, Throat, and Allergy
Roy E. Kerry, M.D.
17 6th Ave.
Greenville, PA 16125
(412) 588-2600

Holistic Health Center
Ralph A. Miranda, M.D.
RD 12, Box 108
Greensburg, PA 15601
(412) 838-7632

Jama Medical Clinic
Donald Mantell, M.D.
6505 Mars Rd.
Cranberry Township, PA 16066
(412) 776-5610

Christiane M. Siewers, M.D.
135 Freeport Rd.
Pittsburgh, PA 15215
(412) 782-4700

Area Code 610
Ferro Chiropractic Wellness
Anthony Ferro, D.C.
2 Pennsbury Way W.
Chadds Ford, PA 19317
(610) 388-2212

Area Code 717
Arthur L. Koch, D.O.
57 W. Juniper St.
Hazleton, PA 18201
(717) 455-4747

George C. Miller II, M.D.
Three Hospital Dr.
Lewisburg, PA 17837
(717) 524-4405

Norman E. Wenger, M.D.
P.O. Box 502
Carbondale, PA 18407
(717) 222-9494

Rhode Island

Area Code 401
Michael C. Rosenberg, D.O.
335 Hope St.
Providence, RI 02906
(401) 272-1832

South Carolina

Area Code 803
Aiken Ear, Nose, Throat & Allergy
Martin Zwerling, M.D.
146 University Pkwy.
Aiken, SC 29801
(803) 648-9555

Biogenesis Medical Center
1000 E. Rutherford Rd.
Landrum, SC 29356
(803) 457-4141

Allan D. Lieberman, M.D.
7510 Northforest Dr.
North Charleston, SC 29420
(803) 572-1600

Area Code 864
Robert G. Mahon, Jr., M.D.
Theodore A. Watson, M.D.
701 Arlington Ave.
Greenville, SC 29601
(864) 233-6881

Tennessee

Area Code 423
Fred M. Furr, M.D.
9217 Park West Blvd.
Bldg. E, Suite 1
Knoxville, TN 37923
(423) 693-1502

Area Code 615
Mitchell & Pitard
Cecil E. Pitard, M.D.
2001 Laurel Ave., #NG2
Knoxville, TN 37916
(615) 522-7714

Donald C. Thompson, M.D.
1121 W. 1st North St.
Morristown, TN 37814
(615) 581-6367

Area Code 901
Richard G. Wanderman, M.D.
5575 Poplar Ave., Suite 112
Memphis, TN 38119
(901) 683-2777

Texas

Area Code 210
Northwest Medical Center
Jim P. Archer, D.O.
8637 Fredericksburg Rd., #150
San Antonio, TX 78240
(210) 697-8445

Area Code 214
Richard G. Jaeckle, M.D.
8220 Walnut Hill Ln., #404
Dallas, TX 75231
(214) 696-0964

R.W. Noble, M.D.
6757 Arapaho Rd., #757
Dallas, TX 75248
(214) 458-9944

William Rea, M.D.
8345 Walnut Hill Ln., Suite 205
Dallas, TX 75231
(214) 368-4132

Gerald H. Ross, M.D.
8345 Walnut Hill Ln., Suite 220
Dallas, TX 75231
(214) 368-4132

Area Code 409
Jody Caldwell, M.D.
1915 N. Frazier
Conroe, TX 77304
(409) 756-3321

Wanda J. Michaels, M.D.
Riceland Regional Mental Health
  Authority
400 Ave. F
Bay City, TX 77414
(409) 245-9231

Area Code 512
Nutrition Counseling Services
James Heffley, Ph.D.
3913 Medical Pkwy., #101
Austin, TX 78756
(512) 453-4051

Russell R. Roby, M.D.
3410 Far West, Suite 110
Austin, TX 78731
(512) 338-4336

Area Code 713
Robert M. Battle, M.D.
9910 Long Point Rd.
Houston, TX 77055
(713) 932-0552

Health Recovery Center
John Parks Trowbridge, M.D.
9816 Memorial Blvd., #205
Humble, TX 77338
(800) FIX-PAIN

Soraya Hoover, M.D.
150 West Parker Rd., Suite 705
Houston, TX 77076
(713) 694-8188

Area Code 806
E. Paul Stewart, M.D.
3812 24th St.
Lubbock, TX 79410
(806) 793-8963

Harlan O. L. Wright, D.O.
4903 82nd St., #50
Lubbock, TX 79424
(806) 794-9632

Area Code 817
Stevan Cordas, D.O.
2921 Brown Trail, #120
Bedford, TX 76021
(817) 498-1679

Utah

Area Code 801
David J. Harbrecht, M.D.
425 Medical Dr., #107
Bountiful, UT 84010
(801) 292-8303

Robert M. Payne, M.D.
166 E. 5900 S., #B111
Murry, UT 84107
(801) 269-8817

Dennis W. Remington, M.D.
1675 N. Freedom Blvd., #11E
Provo, UT 84604
(801) 373-8500

Virginia

Area Code 540
Susan Zimmer, R.N., D.C.
8430 Main St.
P.O. Box 495
Marshall, VA 22115
(540) 364-2045

Area Code 703
Mount Rogers Clinic
Elmer M. Cranton, M.D.
Ripshin Rd.
Trout Dale, VA 24378
(703) 677-3631

Henry J. Palacios, M.D.
1481 Chain Bridge Rd., #101
McLean, VA 22101
(703) 356-2244

Area Code 804
Linwood W. Custalow, M.D.
1832 Todds Ln.
Hampton, VA 23666
(804) 826-0232
(804) 877-9361

Washington

Area Code 206
William R. Bailey, D.O.
515 W. Harrison, Suite 200
Kent, WA 98032
(206) 854-4900

David Buscher, M.D.
1603 116th Ave. N.E., Suite 112
Bellevue, WA 98004
(206) 453-0288

Jenefer S. Huntoon, N.D.
1329 N. 45th St.
Seattle, WA 98103
(206) 632-8804

Davis W. Lamson, N.D., M.S.
515 W. Harrison, Suite 200
Kent, WA 98032
(206) 854-4900

Jonathan V. Wright, M.D.
515 W. Harrison, Suite 200
Kent, WA 98032
(206) 854-4900

Area Code 360
Jonathan Collin, M.D.
911 Tyler St.
Port Townsend, WA 98368
(360) 385-4555
(206) 820-0547 (Kirkland office)

The Fifth Ave. Medical Center
Paul Thompson, M.D.
675 N. 5th Ave.
Sequim, WA 98382
(360) 683-2198

Mount Rainier Clinic, Inc.
Elmer M. Cranton, M.D.
503 First St. S., Suite 1
P.O. Box 7510
Yelm, WA 98597
(360) 458-1061
(800) 337-9918

Laura A. Shelton, N.D.
1707 F St.
Bellingham, WA 98225
(360) 734-1560

Area Code 509
Albert G. Corrado, M.D.
800 Swift, Suite 200
Richland, WA 99352
(509) 946-4631

Yakima Allergy Clinic
302 S. 12th Ave.
Yakima, WA 98902
(509) 453-5507

West Virginia

Area Code 304
Prudencio C. Corro, M.D.
251 Stanaford Rd.
Beckley, WV 25801
(304) 252-0775

Albert V. Jellen, M.D.
2097 National Rd.
Wheeling, WV 26003
(304) 242-5151

Wisconsin

Area Code 414
Eleazar M. Kadile, M.D.
1538 Bellevue St.
Green Bay, WI 54311
(414) 468-9442

Wayne H. Konetzki, M.D.
403 N. Grand Ave.
Waukesha, WI 53186
(414) 547-3055

Area Code 608
Allergy Association of La Crosse
George F. Kroker, M.D.
David L. Morris, M.D.
Mary Morris, M.D.
Vijay Sabnis, M.D.
615 S. 10th St., P.O. Box 2408
La Crosse, WI 54602
(608) 782-2027

Madison Pain & Acupuncture
T. Galvez, M.D.
2705 Marshall Ct.
Madison, WI 53705
(608) 238-3831

Index

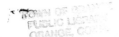